IS ACUPUNCTURE RIGHT FOR YOU?

What It Is, Why It Works, and How It Can Help You

RUTH LEVER KIDSON

Healing Arts Press
Rochester, Vermont

Healing Arts Press
One Park Street
Rochester, Vermont 05767
www.HealingArtsPress.com

Healing Arts Press is a division of Inner Traditions International

Originally published in England in 1987 by Penguin Books Ltd under the title *Acupuncture for Everyone: What It Is, How It Developed, How It Can Help You, and Where to Find Treatment*

First U.S. edition published in 2000 by Healing Arts Press under the title *Acupuncture for Everyone: What It Is, Why It Works, and How It Can Help You*

Second U.S. edition published in 2008 by Healing Arts Press under the title *Is Acupuncture Right for You? What It Is, Why It Works, and How It Can Help You*

Note to the reader: *This book is intended as an informational guide. The remedies, approaches, and techniques described herein are meant to supplement, and not to be a substitute for, professional medical care or treatment. They should not be used to treat a serious ailment without prior consultation with a qualified health care professional.*

Library of Congress Cataloging-in-Publication Data
Kidson, Ruth.
  Is acupuncture right for you? : what it is, why it works, and how it can help you / Ruth Lever Kidson. — 1st U.S. ed.
      p. cm.
  "Originally published in England by Penguin Books."
  Includes bibliographical references and index.
  ISBN 978-1-59477-267-2 (pbk.)
  1. Acupuncture—Popular works. I. Title.
  RM184.K527 2008
  615.8'92—dc22

                                                                            2008027257

Printed and bound in the United States by Lake Book Manufacturing

10 9 8 7 6 5 4 3 2 1

Text design and layout by Carol Ruzicka
This book was typeset in Garamond Premier Pro with Minion as the display typeface

To send correspondence to the author of this book, mail a first-class letter to the author c/o Inner Traditions • Bear & Company, One Park Street, Rochester, VT 05767, and we will forward the communication.

This book is dedicated to the memory of:
Marie Ross and Tom Dummer, who first led me
into the world of complementary medicine;
my aunt, Fredi Morgan; three dear friends,
Rosa Taylor, Margery Lamont, and
Hereward Overnell; and my father, Lionel Lever.

A NOTE ON THE LANGUAGE

Throughout this book doctors, acupuncturists, and patients tend to be referred to as "he." This does not, of course, imply that there are no women doctors, acupuncturists, or patients, but is to prevent the reader from becoming irritated by a constant repetition of "he or she" and to prevent the author from becoming irritated at having to use the ungrammatical "they."

Contents

Introduction

Although it is only in fairly recent times that acupuncture has become a recognized therapy in the West, its popularity as an alternative to Western medicine is increasing, particularly for the treatment of chronically painful conditions. And although of course no therapy—Western or complementary—works for everyone, many patients are finding that acupuncture offers effective relief not just for pain but also for a wide range of medical problems.

Among those patients who have experienced acupuncture and whose health has improved, however, there must be some who have wondered just how much of the improvement was due to the treatment and how much was fortuitous. Did it just happen that their illness took a turn for the better at the same time that they started going to the acupuncturist? Or could it have been a case of mind over matter? Even to those who have experienced acupuncture—and very much more to those who haven't—it can seem a rather bizarre form of treatment. In the tradition of Western medicine we are accustomed to having treatment directed at the part of the body that is malfunctioning. If we sprain an ankle, we have it wrapped; if we develop a boil, we have it lanced; if an appendix becomes inflamed, we have it removed. But acupuncture treats *all* ailments by sticking needles into the skin, and very often the needles are put into areas of the body that seem to be totally unrelated to the illness from which we are suffering.

1

There was a time when people unquestioningly accepted whatever treatment their doctors dished out, but, thankfully, times have changed. Patients nowadays are much better informed and, as a result, are able to play a much more active role in their own recovery from illness. So it is natural that anyone thinking of going to an acupuncturist wants to understand something of the therapy. Cartoons about acupuncture seem always to show someone stuck full of needles looking something like Custer's Last Stand; this perception, together with a lack of accurate knowledge about the therapy, can make the prospect of going for treatment quite frightening. Even in Western medicine a patient will tolerate treatment and investigations far more readily if he is told in advance what is going to be done and why. But nobody likes to appear foolish. It takes a brave patient, already somewhat intimidated by the fact of having things done to him, to speak up and ask, "Why are you doing that? And what do you intend to do next?" The purpose of this book, then, is to explain what the acupuncturist is doing and why.

In order to understand the theory of acupuncture, we have to forget all the concepts of Western medicine that we have been brought up with. Not only is acupuncture theory couched in terms evolved in an alien (Chinese) culture, but it is also far more esoteric than the flesh-and-bones theories of Western medicine. The latter treats the physical matter of the body. If bodily function has become disrupted, Western medicine treats it with drugs—for example, by giving antihypertensives to treat high blood pressure. If a body part has become irreparably diseased or is doing the patient harm, it is surgically removed—for instance, the removal of an inflamed appendix or an overactive thyroid gland. Or if the part has merely become distorted, it may be surgically repaired, as in the case of a prolapsed uterus. For parts of the body whose function is inadequate or inappropriate, there is a variety of therapies whose aim is to encourage the return to normal function, such as physiotherapy for poorly functioning muscles and psychotherapy for mental problems.

Acupuncture, however, uses a single therapy—the insertion of needles into the skin—to treat a variety of ailments that might be treated by Western doctors with drugs, surgery, or a range of other therapies. Acupuncture can treat all ailments in the same way because it sees them as stemming from the same cause—a disruption of the energy flow or vital force of the body. This vital force (of which much more will be said in chapter 2) does not play a role in Western medicine. But in Chinese medicine it is seen as fundamental to normal bodily function; its disruption can result in malfunction and disease. The vital force is said to flow through a system of channels, or meridians, and disruption of that flow will manifest itself as disease in those parts of the body supplied by the affected meridian. The aim of acupuncture, which consists of inserting needles at various well-defined points lying along the meridians, is to restore balance to the energy flow and thus return the associated part to its normal function.

The word *acupuncture* is derived from the Latin *acu* (meaning "with a needle") and the English *puncture,* but in fact piercing the skin is not essential to the treatment. There are several ways in which the flow of energy through the meridians can be manipulated. Indeed, some practitioners prefer to describe the treatment they offer as meridian therapy rather than acupuncture. As an alternative to needles, pressure may be used in a form of massage, or the points may be warmed (or even burned, as I shall mention in chapter 1). Lasers have also been used to stimulate the points. It is nowadays even possible to buy a do-it-yourself acupuncture kit complete with an electrical stimulator with which to treat your own points. However, the latter is not recommended; without thorough training in the theory and practice of acupuncture, it is rather like buying a knife and an anatomy book and trying to take out your own appendix.

This is not, therefore, a teach-yourself-acupuncture book. What I will try to do is to demonstrate how an acupuncturist makes his diagnosis and how, in the light of this diagnosis, he treats his patient. The aim is twofold: to make going to the acupuncturist for the first time less intimidating, and to throw light on some of the mysteries that the therapist may not have time to explain during treatment (such as why, if you go complaining of a headache, he may stick a needle in your foot!).

Acupuncture originated, of course, in a culture quite different from our own and was exported to the West comparatively late in its evolution. Its history, therefore, is a fundamental part of what it is today, and to its history the next chapter is devoted.

1
A Short History of Acupuncture

Acupuncture is based on a completely different set of theories from those of Western medicine. In the West a doctor will base his diagnosis of a patient's illness on his knowledge of anatomy, physiology, biochemistry, and pathology; then, having put a name to the disease, he will decide whether to treat the patient with drugs, surgery, or other techniques. However, there are some patients whom doctors find it very difficult to treat because, although they are clearly unwell, all the tests are normal and a diagnosis cannot be made. For these patients acupuncture (like many other complementary therapies) is perfectly suitable: It does not require a diagnosis in Western terms for the patient to be treated successfully.

Acupuncture is one of the oldest therapies known to humanity, having been in use for well over two thousand years. And although developments have occurred, from time to time, its basic theory and practice are still much the same as when it was practiced twenty centuries ago. This theory also forms the foundation of Chinese herbal medicine, with which acupuncture is frequently used in the East. When acupuncture first became popular in the West it was usually used alone, but many practitioners now train in herbal medicine as well so that they can offer both therapies.

The oldest-known book on the theory of Chinese medicine is the *Nei Ching,* which has been published in English under the title *The Yellow Emperor's Classic of Internal Medicine.* It is written in the form of a

5

dialogue, the two participants being Huang Ti (the Yellow Emperor) and Ch'i Po, a Taoist teacher and physician. (In ancient times physicians were often religious teachers as well, in much the same way that many Western monks were highly skilled in herbal medicine.)

The Yellow Emperor is said to have lived in the twenty-seventh century B.C. In fact, there is disagreement among scholars as to whether he lived at all or was just a mythical character—perhaps one originally based on a real person who, over the centuries, has been endowed with far more greatness than he actually warranted. It is rather like the arguments that take place in Britain as to whether there really was a King Arthur. However, even if the Yellow Emperor was a real person, it is highly unlikely that the *Nei Ching* in its present form can be attributed to him or even dated to his reign.

In the twenty-seventh century B.C. written Chinese was still in a fairly primitive form known as archaic, or prehistoric, ideographs. The *Nei Ching* is an extremely profound work, and it would have been impossible for much of it to have been expressed in this primitive script. The most recent thinking is that the *Nei Ching* is made up of several different treatises, possibly originating from particular medical theorists or schools. It is felt that these treatises were written at different times between about 200 B.C. and A.D. 100, and then put together at the end of this period. This, of course, still makes it a work of considerable antiquity.

However, although the *Nei Ching* is the oldest book on Chinese medicine that has come down to us, it was unlikely to have been the first book ever written on the subject. It was not written in a way that suggests it is introducing something new and original. Indeed, by the time it was written, acupuncture was obviously widely understood and practiced in China. The *Nei Ching* gives the reader no instructions whatsoever on basic theory or on the points and techniques to be used—it is assumed that he already knows these. The book covers only the more esoteric aspects of theory, such as "the transmission of the essence and the transmission of the life-giving principle" and "the seasons as patterns of the viscera." The Yellow Emperor asks questions, which are then answered at length by Ch'i Po. Some of the questions are very profound, running to several pages, and among the things that Ch'i Po is asked to explain are "how it is possible that the twelve viscera send each other that which is precious and that which is worthless" and "whether the brain and the marrow govern the viscera or whether it is the stomach that governs the viscera, or whether the viscera govern the six bowels." The Yellow Emperor—real or mythical—obviously had a very good grasp of the basic theories of Chinese medicine!

Stories of great acupuncturists have also come down to us from two thousand or more years ago. A century or two before the *Nei Ching* is thought to have been written, although somewhat after the time of the Yellow Emperor himself, there lived a famous itinerant Chinese physician and teacher of medicine called Pien Chueh. His actual dates are unknown but, traditionally, he is said to have lived in the fourth century B.C. One story told about him describes a time when he was visiting the province of Kuo with some of his students, or apprentices. Upon reaching the town in which the king and his court resided, they saw many sacrifices being offered at the temples and arrangements being made for a funeral. When Pien Chueh asked what was happening he was told that the king's son had suddenly fallen ill and lapsed into a coma from which the court physicians had been unable to rouse him. It seemed inevitable that he would die. Pien Chueh asked his informant whether he could arrange for him to be introduced at court; he thought he might be able to prevent the boy from dying. Arrangements were made accordingly, and the king willingly allowed Pien Chueh to examine the comatose prince.

After a thorough examination Pien Chueh made a diagnosis based on his extensive knowledge of Chinese medicine. He then treated the prince, placing acupuncture needles in his head, chest, arms, and legs, after which the boy rapidly regained consciousness. Pien Chueh continued to treat him and monitor his progress for three weeks. In addition to acupuncture, he used heat treatment and herbal remedies. At the end of this period the prince was restored to full health. What happened to the court physicians the story does not tell, but it is possible that the king made arrangements for them to learn the basics of acupuncture!

The description of Pien Chueh using heat to treat his patient may be referring to moxibustion, a method—still in use today—in which the acupuncture points are stimulated by heat. The name derives from an herb known as moxa, which is burned to supply the heat. Nowadays the usual practice is to attach a small wad of moxa to the end of an acupuncture needle that has already been inserted into the patient; when this is lit the heat travels down the needle and into the point without running the risk of burning the skin. Originally, however, the custom was to put the moxa directly onto the skin or on a slice of ginger placed over the relevant acupuncture point, and this latter method is still used by some practitioners. How moxibustion fits into the chronology of acupuncture is uncertain. Some people think it may predate acupuncture, since some ancient texts have been found that mention moxa but not acupuncture. Although these particular texts were found in a tomb that dates back to the Han dynasty (206 B.C.–A.D. 220—a time during which, as we know from other sources, acupuncture was already widely used), they may have been copies of others that were considerably older. And although moxa has been used therapeutically for many centuries, the healing quality of warmth applied to the acupuncture points was probably known long before the burning properties of moxa leaves were discovered and before needles were used to treat the points. Perhaps twigs and grass were originally used to produce a similar effect. Records show that various other substances, such as charcoal, bamboo, and sulfur, have all been used in the past.

The dried moxa leaves, when burned, smell not unlike cannabis—or so I was once told by a teenage patient, who informed me that my consulting room smelled like a rock concert! Moxa, like cannabis or that other dried leaf of ill repute, tobacco, has the ability to burn slowly and steadily. It is used primarily to treat diseases said to have been caused by cold or damp (I will discuss this in depth in chapter 4). And although it was, and still is, often found to be useful in its homeland of China, it has been used to a far greater extent in Japan. Being made up of islands, Japan tends to have a much more humid climate than the great expanse of China, so its incidence of diseases associated with damp is much greater. It is therefore appropriate that the name by which this treatment is known in the West—*moxa*—should, in fact, be Japanese in origin, derived from two words that mean "burning herb." The Chinese name for moxa is *chiu*, which means "to cauterize or blister."

It has been suggested that the accidental burning of acupuncture points may have led to the discovery of their therapeutic value. Acupuncture is such an ancient therapy that its origins are completely unknown. Strangely, in view of China's many ancient myths and folk heroes, there is not even, as far as I know, any legend explaining how it originated. The burn theory is one of several that has been put forward. It suggests that in the days when people huddled around fires that served the dual purpose of keeping them warm and cooking their food, it is likely that they were frequently burned by sparks flying out from the fire. If a spark landed on, and a burn subsequently occurred on, an appropriate acupuncture point, people may have been "miraculously" cured of various illnesses that had been troubling them. After this had happened on a number of occasions and to a number of people, they might have started to realize that in some way these particular points on the body had healing properties. In some patients stimulation of a single point will cause a sensation to run along the meridian on which it lies. In other patients, you can sometimes see a flush spreading along the line of the meridian when a point is needled. Based on this, the early Chinese could have started to work out a system of lines that joined the points together—the predecessors of the meridians that we know today. And of course it would appear to them that the way in which to use these points therapeutically was to burn them, since it was through burning that the effects seemed to arise. This, then, ties in with the point I made earlier: that moxa treatment of the acupuncture points may well have developed before acupuncture itself.

Another theory concerning the origin of acupuncture is that, in the days when there was constant warring between neighboring tribes, men who were wounded in battle may have found that injuries inflicted in certain spots had a therapeutic effect on various diseases from which they were suffering. This is a theory much loved by cartoonists, who depict men lying on the battlefield, run through with spears or stuck full of arrows, making such comments as, "That's done wonders for my hay fever."

Other possibilities may seem more feasible. I have heard it suggested that the earliest therapists were healers who used the "laying on of hands" method common all over the world. Healers nowadays often say that they feel a sensation in their hands—cold, heat, or tingling—when they have their hands over an area of the patient's body that is in need of treatment. It is possible that these early healers may have been particularly sensitive and intuitive and thus able to pick up the position of acupuncture points that needed treating, developing the theory of the meridians from there. According to another theory, the treatment may originally have involved piercing the skin in a fairly random way to drive out devils whose presence in the body was thought to be the cause of illness. Eventually it might have been possible for those performing the treatment to work out which points were effective for which types of illness and, from there, to develop the more elaborate theories of acupuncture.

A fascinating and fairly recent discovery is that acupuncture was not confined to China in its earliest days. In 1991 the body of a man was found ten thousand feet up a glacier on the northern border of Italy. He had died some five thousand years ago and been perfectly preserved by the ice. Upon examination he was found to have been suffering from an arthritic condition that would have caused him pain in his back and hips. His skin showed strange tattoos over the diseased joints and on his feet. Upon further investigation these appeared to be at the sites of acupuncture points. Acupuncturist Dr. Frank Bahr was asked his opinion. If a patient presented to him with the arthritic problems of this man, Dr. Bahr said, the points he would use in treatment would correspond 90 percent to the points marked by the tattoos. Bahr suggested that the tattooing was a form of "doctor's letter"—a message from one practitioner to another indicating which points should be used to treat the patient.

If this is indeed the case—that acupuncture was being used in Europe five thousand years ago—we have an additional conundrum. Not only do we not know how and why acupuncture developed, but we are also unclear why it stood the test of time in China but died out elsewhere. It seems unlikely that we shall ever find out.

What we can be fairly sure of, however, is that once the acupuncture points were discovered—by whatever means—the next stage would have been to experiment with different methods of stimulating them. The earliest acupuncture tools seem to have been sharp pieces of stone or flint, which were known as bian stones. Their use would have been limited because of their size and shape, so they were probably used just to scratch, or possibly to prick, the points on the meridian. Sharp pieces of pottery were also used. The next instruments to be developed were somewhat more versatile: They were made from sharpened bones and bamboo, which could be formed into a more needlelike shape. However, it was not until the smelting of metal had been discovered that it was possible to manufacture true needles that could be inserted through the patient's skin and into the layers below.

The earliest needles were made from various types of metals as they became available—iron, bronze, silver, and even gold. Silver and gold acupuncture needles have been found in the tomb of Prince Liu Sheng, who lived and died during the Western Han dynasty (206 B.C. through A.D. 24). Given this inclusion in burial goods, it would seem that the people of the period thought that, even in heaven, their health might need attention!

Since metal was so much more versatile than the stones, bones, and bamboo that had previously been used, it became possible to develop different shapes of needles, which could then be used for different techniques. These may originally have been made by chance since, presumably, the earliest metalsmithing was a fairly crude affair that could not be expected to produce identical needles every time. Presented with these varying shapes, however, the early acupuncture practitioners may have realized that different-shaped needles produced different effects. Therefore, as the quality of the smithing improved, they would have ordered the specific shapes that they found most useful.

When the *Nei Ching* was written some two thousand years ago, nine types of needles were already in common use, not unlike the variety of needles still in use today. There were fine needles, which (as now) were used for the majority of straightforward treatments. There were arrowhead needles, which were used when it was necessary only to prick the point, rather than to insert a needle. To induce slight bleeding at a point, three-sided needles were available. Needles with a triangular tip terminating in a sharp point are still used today when bleeding is required. Blunt or round-ended needles were used when points needed pressure or massaging, and scalpel-like needles were used for incising boils and abscesses. Larger, heavier needles were available for inserting into joints. Extra-long needles were used when the most receptive part of the acupuncture point lay well below the skin surface in an area of thick muscle or fat. Today needles up to three inches long are used in areas such as the buttocks, but even these are considerably shorter than some said to have been used by the early acupuncturists.

The majority of needles used in acupuncture practice today are made of stainless steel, which was first developed in the early years of the twentieth century. Its great advantages are that it can easily be sterilized and will not rust. However, since the appearance of AIDS and the various forms of hepatitis that can be transmitted through blood, more and more acupuncturists are working with disposable needles, which are used once only and then thrown away.

Before stainless steel was developed, however, silver and gold needles were quite widely used, because these two metals are relatively inert and less likely to cause unwanted reactions when inserted into patients. There may have been other reasons for their popularity: It was thought that gold needles had, of themselves, a stimulating effect (this was also said to be true of the other yellow metal, copper), while silver and other white metal needles had a calming effect. Today needles made of precious metals have definite disadvantages in that they are much more expensive than stainless steel; too valuable to be thrown away when they become blunt, they must be resharpened. Some practitioners are still sufficiently convinced of their intrinsic therapeutic effects to go on using them, though. A letter was published in the December 1985 *American Journal of Acupuncture* from a doctor in Spain who had found that, when he was treating patients for pain, he obtained the best results by using gold needles for patients whose pain was made worse by movement or those whose pain was due to inflammation or disuse. Silver needles were best when the pain was due to overuse of the part concerned.

In the same way that Western medical students learn both general medicine and surgery as part of their basic curriculum, herbal medicine (based on the same fundamental theories of body function and energy flow as acupuncture) has always been taught in China alongside acupuncture. And as you might expect with such ancient therapies, the earliest recorded medical schools were founded centuries before those in the West. The first state-sponsored school in China to teach all aspects of Chinese medicine opened in A.D. 443 but was closed again within ten years. Student physicians had to revert to the traditional method of learning—apprenticeship to an experienced doctor. In A.D. 581, during the Sui dynasty, an Imperial Medical Academy was founded. However, it was under the following Tang dynasty (618–906) that medical education really started to develop. In A.D. 624 the academy was greatly enlarged. Departments were set up to teach pharmacology, acupuncture, internal medicine, and massage—as well as Buddhist and Taoist incantation, which at the time were thought essential knowledge for a physician. For the first time it became possible to study acupuncture and moxibustion as disciplines separate from herbal medicine.

The length of training required to become a physician was as long as or longer than that required in the West today. Before a student was allowed to specialize in any one aspect of medicine, he had to take a general basic course. When he had passed this, he was allowed to study internal medicine, which took a further seven years; or surgery, which took five years; or pediatrics, which also took five years. Less time was required to train in more limited specialties such as diseases of the ear, nose, and throat.

Like medical schools today, the Imperial Medical Academy taught from standard textbooks. The *Nei Ching* was, of course, one of them. Another was Huang-Pu Mi's *Chia I Ching* (The Classic of Acupuncture

Fundamentals), which was written in the third century A.D. and is the oldest-known book of its kind, being devoted entirely to acupuncture and moxibustion. Many later books used the *Chia I Ching* as a source, and it played an important role in the development of acupuncture in Japan and Korea. A third standard text in use at the Imperial Medical Academy was Wang Su-Ho's *Mai Ching* (The Classic of the Pulse).

Pulse taking is a much more exact and detailed science in Chinese medicine than it is in the West, and it plays a far more important role in diagnosis. (I will discuss it in some depth in chapter 5.) It may take a student many years to become an expert in interpreting the pulse. And because not just acupuncture but all forms of traditional Chinese medicine are based on the same theories of the causation of disease, pulse diagnosis is fundamental to them all. Wang Su-Ho's *Classic of the Pulse* was not expounding a newly developed science but was compiled from ancient diagnostic techniques that had grown up alongside Chinese medicine as it developed. Other books, published long before Wang Su-Ho's, had mentioned pulse diagnosis—including, of course, the *Nei Ching,* which gives some quite detailed descriptions of the quality of the pulse in different disease states. The great fourth-century acupuncturist Pien Chueh, whom we have already met in the story of his treatment of the comatose prince of Kuo, is known to have used pulse diagnosis. It may, of course, have been his ability as a diagnostician, rather than his skills in treatment, that enabled him to treat the prince successfully when the court physicians had failed.

Pien Chueh is said to have been the first physician to use together the four basic techniques of Chinese diagnosis. The first of these is *observation,* in which the physician looks at his patient's complexion, color, skin, and tongue in much the same way that a Western physician does today—although of course his findings would be interpreted differently, according to traditional Chinese theory. The tongue, like the pulse, can tell a traditionally trained Chinese physician far more than it can a Western doctor, and its observation is an important method of diagnosis. (This too is described more fully in chapter 5.) The physician also observes his patient's expression as an aid to diagnosis. The second technique, or group of techniques, used by Pien Chueh comprised *listening and smelling*. He would listen to the quality of the patient's speech—normal, slurred, high pitched, and so on—and to the sound of his breathing, although of course he lacked the benefit of that modern Western tool the stethoscope. He would also smell the patient's body odors—probably more important in a society where hot and cold running water were unknown and baths were probably taken infrequently. This technique is still used by some acupuncture practitioners, however, and is even occasionally of use in current Western medicine. For example, the smell of acetone on a patient's breath is accepted as a clear indication that he is a diabetic whose condition is getting out of control. The third technique on Pien Chueh's list was *questioning,* which of course plays an important role in all forms of medicine—Western, Chinese, and other complementary therapies. Finally, he would use *pulse diagnosis.*

The Classic of the Pulse was exported to Japan and Korea in the sixth century A.D. Chinese medicine had reached both countries several centuries earlier, and techniques of pulse diagnosis were rapidly assimilated into their medical practice. The *Chu Ping Yuan Hou Lun* (A Discourse on the Causes and Symptoms of All Illnesses), published only a few years later in A.D. 610 was also to become extremely influential in the development of Japanese and Korean medicine. Its grandiose title was perhaps justified, since it stretched to fifty volumes and compiled virtually all the medical knowledge of the time. Its editor was Chao Yuan Fang, a physician at the imperial court.

As Chinese medicine developed during the Tang dynasty its fame spread, and soon physicians from other nations were arriving in China to learn new techniques. Arabian doctors came to learn the art of pulse diagnosis and to study infectious diseases. *The Classic of the Pulse* was exported to the Middle East some time in the eleventh century, and by the mid-fourteenth century it had been translated into Turkish. The great Persian physician Abu-Ali al-Husain ibn Abdullah ibn Sina, better known as Avicenna (980–1037), wrote an immense work in Arabic called *Al-Qanun fi'l-Tibb* (The Canon of Medicine) in which he discussed the medical achievements of the great Greek physicians and described medical techniques that had been written about in other Arabic works. To this he added information about the methods that he himself had developed during his own years of practice, based on what he had been taught during his travels and what he had learned from reading. Among these was pulse diagnosis. Avicenna recorded twenty-four different types of pulse of which he was aware.

During the Sung dynasty (960–1279) acupuncture and moxibustion became very popular in China, mainly due to the patronage of the nobility and the emperors. But despite this, and despite the fact that acupuncture and the diagnostic techniques of Chinese medicine were now becoming familiar in other parts of Asia and in the Middle East, the Chinese imperial court felt that over the years inaccuracies had arisen in the practice of this therapy. Many of the early books on acupuncture had been lost, and many of the standard reference books were compilations into which errors could have crept. In the eleventh century Wang Wei-I—the court physician to two of the emperors of the Northern Sung dynasty, Chen-Tsung (997–1022) and Jen-Tsung (1022–1063)—was instructed to investigate the validity of the system of acupuncture that was currently being practiced and to carry out what would be the first major revision of acupuncture theory.

Wang Wei-I embarked on a mammoth research program. He investigated all the acupuncture points that were currently being used and verified their locations. He also studied each point in turn and confirmed to what depth each should be punctured in order to produce an effect. Finally, he identified the effects that might be produced by the needling of each point. He published his findings in a book titled *The New Illustrated Manual on the Points for Acupuncture*.

Wang Wei-I's exact dates are unknown; he may well have died before 1034, which was the year in which his imperial patron, Emperor Jen-Tsung, was taken ill. The emperor, who was an orthodox Confucian and a patron of scholars, was twenty-two years old at the time and had been attended by imperial physicians who, using methods other than acupuncture, had been unable to cure him. Eventually he was successfully treated with acupuncture by a highly skilled practitioner named Xu Xi. However, the courtiers in attendance on the emperor nearly prevented the treatment from taking place. After examining the patient, Xu Xi let it be known that he proposed to insert acupuncture needles into the emperor's chest, just below the level of his heart. The courtiers were horrified and said that on no account must the treatment take place; far from curing the emperor, it would no doubt kill him. Xu Xi assured them that the treatment was quite safe and offered to demonstrate the technique on someone whose death, if it occurred, would be less of a disaster. This proposition was acceptable to the courtiers, and it was decided that he could demonstrate on the court eunuchs, who were presumably expendable. Xu Xi inserted his needles into the eunuchs at the point he had described, and the courtiers were amazed and relieved to find that he had spoken the truth: The eunuchs were unharmed. (No doubt the eunuchs were even more relieved!) Xu Xi was therefore allowed to return to the emperor's presence and treat him in the manner that he had demonstrated. Fortunately for both Xu Xi and the emperor, the latter made a rapid recovery. Everyone at court was so impressed by this demonstration of skill that Xu Xi was appointed medical officer of the Imperial Medical Academy.

Although it seems that some of the court physicians attendant on Jen-Tsung were not particularly adept at acupuncture, Wang Wei-I, who served both him and Emperor Chen-Tsung, is still remembered for the contribution he made both to the treatment itself and to its teaching. He used a model of a man cast in bronze, the surface of which was punctured with holes accurately placed at the positions of all the acupuncture points. This was, of course, based on all the research that he had undertaken when compiling his *New Illustrated Manual on the Points for Acupuncture*. Wang Wei-I's bronze men became valuable teaching aids for students of acupuncture, and were also used to test their knowledge in examinations held at the Imperial Medical Academy. Before the exam the model was covered with a thick layer of wax, which was then allowed to set so that the holes at the position of the acupuncture points could not be seen. The hollow interior of the model was then filled with water. A student would be told about a case and asked how he would treat it using acupuncture. After describing which points he would use and why, he was asked to locate them on the model and told to insert a needle into each of them, through the wax. If he located the points accurately, the needles would go through the wax and into the holes below so that, when the needles were removed, water would flow out.

In the mid-sixteenth century, five hundred years after Wang Wei-I cast his first bronze model, his idea was developed even further by an acupuncturist named Kao Wu. Wang Wei-I's figures had all been of men, but Kao Wu thought it important to demonstrate that the location of acupuncture points differed according to the sex and age of the patient. He therefore had bronze figures cast of women and children, which could be used in the same way as Wang Wei-I's bronze men.

Kao Wu believed that many errors had arisen in acupuncture practice since Wang Wei-I had carried out his great investigation, and he set himself the task of rectifying this. He wrote two important books on the subject. The first, *Essentials of Acupuncture and Moxibustion,* was a summary of earlier major acupuncture works intended as a guide for students of acupuncture who were just embarking on their studies. His other great work, *Eminent Acupuncture,* was for more advanced students and qualified practitioners. It gave detailed information about the meridians and the points and how they should be used in the treatment of a variety of diseases.

Like Kao Wu's *Essentials of Acupuncture and Moxibustion,* many other "new" acupuncture books were being written around this time that simply revised and summarized the works of earlier authors. However, in 1601 the acupuncturist Yang Jizhou published *A Compendium of Acupuncture and Moxibustion.* Here he not only summarized what had been written about acupuncture in previous centuries but also included a large amount of information based on the results of his own research and experience. As an "original," this book was a great success both in China and in the other countries in Asia to which the practice of acupuncture had spread.

By this time acupuncture and traditional Chinese medicine were being used far beyond the borders of China. In some countries, such as Japan and Korea, they had become the accepted form of medical treatment. Chinese medicine had first been introduced into these two countries many centuries before, during the Chin dynasty (249–206 B.C.), but it was with the spread of Buddhism that it really began to gain popularity. Buddhism, which originated in India in the sixth century B.C., reached China sometime around the middle of the first century A.D. There it developed in tradition and practice and, in the second half of the fourth century, was introduced into Korea. Some two hundred years later it spread to Japan, where the Zen school (which today has followers all around the world) developed. Although Buddhism was not an immediate success among the Japanese people, the regent Shotoku Taishi (593–622) was converted and began to encourage Buddhist monks to come to Japan from China.

In China Buddhist monks often studied Chinese medicine and acupuncture. During the Sui (589–618) and Tang dynasties many of these physician-monks came to Japan. While they were there, they taught the Japanese whatever they wished to learn—not just Buddhist doctrine but also the fundamentals of Chinese medicine.

All the early Buddhist texts had been written in Pali but, with the spread of the religion, more scriptures were written in Sanskrit and in Chinese, and earlier works were translated. It took time before translations could be prepared for a newly converted country, however, so all the texts being used by the monks who went to Japan were in Chinese. If the Japanese converts wanted to read the original scriptures and not just hear about them from the monks (who, no doubt, were adding their own interpretations to them), they would have to learn to read Chinese. And this is what many of them did. Of course, having become proficient in Chinese, they could then read not only the scriptures but also all the texts from which the monks had been teaching them the essentials of medicine and acupuncture. During the seventh century young Japanese men started to go to China to learn the language, and many came back with knowledge not just of Chinese but of Chinese medicine as well.

Once enough Japanese physicians were fluent in the Chinese language, translations could be made of the major Chinese medical texts so that they would be available to all. The *Nei Ching* was one of the first to be translated; by the beginning of the eighth century it was one of the standard textbooks for Japanese medical students. Large numbers of Chinese medical books were brought to Japan in the mid-eighth century by a man named Chien-Chen, who was both a physician and a philanthropist. He established a charity clinic in Japan for the treatment of the poor. Centuries later his memory was still being venerated in Japanese temples as a result of his work with the sick and needy.

Chinese medicine remained popular in Japan until the sixteenth century, when it became overshadowed by influences from the West. This was the period of the great trading companies, with ships being sent from Europe to build up markets and find suppliers of luxuries in far-flung places around the world. The Portuguese, who were ardent believers in the superiority of Roman Catholicism over all "pagan" religions, sent ships to the Far East with more in mind than mere trading. Initially, the reception they received was hostile, since it was discovered that they were prepared to trade only with people whom they could not vanquish. Weaker communities ran the risk of being overrun and massacred. However, after being allowed access to only one town in the whole of China (and that being one with which they had to trade), the second wave of this Portuguese invasion was somewhat gentler, consisting of a number of missionaries who were able to gain a foothold in both China and Japan. Like the Buddhist monks who had come to Japan in the sixth century, these missionaries had some knowledge of medicine—although this was, of course, the comparatively primitive medicine being practiced in Europe at the time. But because it was new and different, or perhaps because of the forceful personalities of those who brought it to the East, it usurped the practice of traditional Chinese medicine in Japan.

Over the next three centuries acupuncture and Chinese medicine were still practiced in Japan, but they played second fiddle to Western medicine. In 1884 an attempt was made to wipe them out completely when an edict prohibiting the teaching of acupuncture and herbal medicine anywhere in the country was issued to coincide with the founding of the medical facility of Tokyo University. Not even this, however, could stop people from practicing the therapies in which they believed. Up to the present day traditional medicine and acupuncture have continued to be used alongside Western techniques.

Surprisingly, in 1822—sixty-two years before the teaching of acupuncture and Chinese medicine was prohibited in Japan—their use was banned in their homeland, China, by Ch'ing dynasty emperor Tao Kuang. The subjects were removed from the syllabus of the Imperial Medical Academy, but (as was to happen later in Japan) their use could not be stopped, since the people were aware of their value and would not give them up.

In 1912 the Imperial dynasty was overthrown and replaced by the radical Kuomintang party, who ruled China until the end of the Second World War when they in turn were ousted by the Communists. The Communists, aware of the people's views concerning acupuncture and traditional Chinese medicine, removed the prohibitions on their use. Indeed, acupuncture was actively encouraged and allowed to flourish. Many of the ancient Chinese medical books that had been used over the centuries as standard texts were reprinted, and many new books were written. Colleges specializing in the teaching of traditional Chinese medicine were set up, all with separate departments of acupuncture. Research institutes were founded for the investigation of acupuncture and the furtherance of its practice. In the existing medical schools—which, since the ban of 1822, had taught nothing but Western medicine—acupuncture found its way back into the curriculum. China now has many medical schools, and since 1949 acupuncture has been taught in all of them in an integrated course alongside Western medicine.

In a number of Asian countries acupuncture remains a popular therapy. In Vietnam, where it was introduced during the Han dynasty, a system has grown up in recent years whereby patients who are admitted to a hospital are treated with Western techniques, but acupuncture and traditional herbal medicine are used for everyday ills.

It is perhaps surprising that Western medicine—which until around the turn of this century was a fairly crude discipline with little to offer in the way of curative techniques—should have so easily superseded the practice of the far more sophisticated Chinese medicine and acupuncture in the Far East, particularly in Japan and China. Maybe it says something about the willingness of the Chinese and Japanese to accept new ideas compared with Westerners: Although acupuncture was introduced into Europe during the seventeenth century, at roughly the same time that Western medicine was having such an impact in the East, it did not attain popularity among Westerners until the second half of the twentieth century. This may be due to the fact that when Western medicine was introduced to the East it was still in its infancy, and so the Chinese and Japanese could learn about its development gradually: acupuncture, however, was already a highly developed therapy and (to the Western mind) very hard to understand by the time it was introduced into Europe.

Interest in acupuncture really only developed in the West when it was realized that it could be used in place of anesthetics for controlling pain during operations. The effectiveness of acupuncture in relieving pain caused by disease had, of course, been known for centuries in the countries where it was practiced. However, surgery started to be performed on a large scale only at the end of the nineteenth century, and it wasn't until 1958 that Chinese doctors began to use acupuncture to control postoperative pain. The results they obtained were so good that they decided to see whether it was possible to control the pain of a minor operation—tonsillectomy was the first to be tried—without having to use any other form of anesthesia. Again, the results were excellent, and they began to use acupuncture for other minor operations such as tooth extractions and the repair of hernias. Although they found that not all patients treated with acupuncture developed a sufficient degree of anesthesia to allow it to be used as the sole method of pain control during an operation, many patients were able to tolerate surgery without any other form of anesthetic. Nowadays even major operations are performed regularly in China's hospitals using only acupuncture to stop the pain. Of course, the advantages of this are enormous: All the risks and unpleasant side effects associated with drug-induced anesthesia are avoided.

As I have noted, acupuncture was first introduced into Europe at least by the seventeenth century, by men who had traveled to China under the auspices of the great trading companies. One of the first European countries to show an interest in acupuncture was France, and one of the earliest books to be written on acupuncture by a European was by the Frenchman Placide Harvieu (1671–1746). It was splendidly titled *The Secrets of Chinese Medicine and the Perfect Knowledge of the Pulse, Brought from China by a Respected Frenchman*. Soon afterward, another book on acupuncture was published in France written by the Reverend Father Cleyer—who presumably did not intend to appeal to a wide audience, since he wrote it in Latin.

A Dutchman, Willem ten Rhyne (1649–1700), practiced acupuncture in Java and also wrote on the subject, but it was the French Dr. Louis-Joseph Berlioz (1776–1848) who was probably the first European actually to practice acupuncture in the West. Sadly, his pioneering work is scarcely remembered; the name *Berlioz* is associated in most people's minds only with his famous son, the composer Hector Berlioz. However, Dr. Berlioz left behind him a book, *Memoirs on Chronic Complaints,* which he had had published in 1816 and in which he devoted a chapter to the practice of acupuncture. In the following decade several books were published in France on the subject, including J. Morand's *Dissertation sur l'acupuncture et ses effets therapeutiques* (1825), Jean Baptiste Sarlandiere's *Memoires sur l'electro-puncture, consideree comme moyen nouveau de traiter efficacement la goutte, les rhumatismes et les affections nerveuses, et sur l'emploi du moxa japonais en France; suivis d'un traite de l'acupuncture et du moxa, principaux moyens curatifs chez les peuples de la Chine, de la Coree et du Japon* (1825), and Jules Cloquet's *Traite de l'acupuncture* (1826), while in London in 1821 James Morss Churchill published *A treatise on acupuncturation: being a description of a surgical operation originally peculiar to the Japonese and Chinese, and by them denominated zin-king, now introduced into European practice, with directions for its performance, and cases illustrating its success.*

In Italy Francesco Rizzoli (1809–1880), who was professor of surgery at Bologna and an outstanding and innovative surgeon, was using acupressure (but not acupuncture) as early as 1854. Ten years later Sir James Young Simpson (1811–1870), who was a professor of obstetrics at Edinburgh and is mainly remembered as the first person to use chloroform in midwifery, published *Acupressure: A New Method of Arresting Surgical Haemorrhage and of Accelerating the Healing of Wounds.* However, despite the fact that some Western physicians were interested enough in acupuncture and acupressure to investigate them, write about them, and in a few cases even practice them, the interest did not spread among the rest of the profession.

In the early years of the twentieth century Georges Soulie de Morant, who resided in China as the representative of a French bank, decided to study acupuncture himself. At the end of his studies he was awarded the title Master Physician. He remained in China for twenty years, eventually becoming the French consul, and during this time he translated into French several works on Chinese medicine as well as writing two books of his own. Of these, *The Synopsis of the True Chinese Acupuncture* was published in 1934, and *Acupuncture* was published in two volumes in 1939.

The main center of interest, such as it was, remained in France. In that country a modern offshoot of acupuncture, auriculotherapy, was developed by Dr. Thomas Nogier, who published *A Treatise of Auriculotherapy* in 1972. In this system needles are inserted into the ear, which is said to reflect the body in microcosm, with specific points being associated with different parts of the body—a lung point, a stomach point, a knee point, and so on. If a disease is localized, the patient can be treated by having needles inserted into the appropriate points.

In Germany the theory of acupuncture was first introduced at the end of the seventeenth century by Engelbert Kaempfer, a naturalist and traveler who devoted two chapters of his *History of Japan* to the subject. In 1906, at a time when the establishment of a Chinese medicine research institute in Germany was sparking the publication of many new books on traditional Chinese medicine and acupuncture in the German language, Kaempfer's book was translated into English but had little impact in Britain. It was not until 1958 that a group of British doctors went to Germany to investigate the use of acupuncture. Their interest may have been stimulated by a paper published the previous year in *The Lancet* by Dr. Louis Moss, a London general practitioner, who reported the results of the treatment of some two thousand patients suffering from arthritis. Dr. Moss found that treatment of certain "trigger points" gave these patients permanent relief from pain, and he noted that these points tallied well with the position of certain acupuncture points.

In the United States and Canada acupuncture and traditional Chinese medicine arrived with the Chinese people, who settled here from the early nineteenth century onward. But these people tended to remain within their own communities, and their customs and therapies spread little to the rest of the population. Still, there was some interest in the subject and a few books were published, such as *The Chinese Way of Medicine* by Edward Hume in 1940 and a partial translation of the *Nei Ching* by Ilza Veith in 1949. Although Dr. Veith's skill in the Chinese language enabled her to produce a readable and informative translation of this very difficult work, it is obvious that she had had no personal experience of acupuncture when she started work on the book. In the introduction she wrote, "Even the practice of acupuncture and moxibustion has survived, despite the fact that these treatments must be exceedingly painful to the patient"—clear indication that she had never even seen a patient being treated with acupuncture. In fact, in the preface to the revised 1965 edition of the book she wrote that "at the time of the . . . publication of this work, the subject of my study seemed to be entirely esoteric."

In the past two decades acupuncture has grown enormously in popularity in the West. It was probably first brought into public awareness by President Nixon's visit to China in 1972. In both Britain and the United States there must be few large towns left that do not have at least one acupuncturist. The therapy, together with Chinese herbal medicine, has received quite a lot of coverage in the popular press and on television during the past few years. There are established training colleges that teach both acupuncture and traditional Chinese medicine and a number of English-language journals for practitioners. Indeed, these therapies have become so well accepted that the London School of Acupuncture and Traditional Chinese Medicine has become part of the University of Westminster, its three-year training course leading to a bachelor of science degree.

2

Fundamental Principles

HOLISM

Acupuncture, as it has been used over the centuries by the Chinese, can truly be described as a holistic therapy. Many people, however, have become confused as to what is actually meant by the word *holistic*—which has been bandied around quite a bit in recent years, particularly when complementary (non-Western) therapies are under discussion.

The word *holism* seems to have been coined in the 1920s by Jan Smuts to mean, in the words of the *Oxford English Dictionary,* "the tendency in nature to produce wholes from the ordered grouping of units." Sometimes you will see it spelled *wholism,* but since Smuts derived it from the Greek word *holos* (meaning "whole") and not from the English word *whole,* it is more correct to spell it without a *w.* Thus *holistic* means "encompassing the whole" and, in terms of medicine, implies the treatment of the patient as a whole. It is not synonymous with *complementary* or *alternative* when referring to therapies, because, although most complementary therapies are holistic when properly used, it is perfectly possible to use most, if not all, of them in a nonholistic way.

In recent years the idea of holism has crept into the Western medical world, with medical practitioners in the United States and Britain forming their own holistic medical associations. Much of holism resides in the attitude of the therapist toward his patient and so, in the same way that it is possible for complementary therapies to be practiced in a nonholistic way, it is perfectly possible for a Western practitioner to practice holistically by taking account of all his patient's problems and relating them to the patient as a whole. Indeed, this was the strength of the old-fashioned family doctor compared with today's overworked general practitioner. The family doctor knew each of his patients individually; he knew their parents, their husbands or wives, and their children, because all of them would have been his patients too. He knew where his patients worked, the sort of food that they could afford, and the kind of housing they lived in. He was a part of the community—he lived in the same town or village as his patients and got to know them socially. When he made a house call to visit one patient, he would probably be given a chance to speak to other members of the family, many of whom would be living nearby. It was therefore a great deal easier for him to see the patient as a whole than it is for a general practitioner today, whose patients often live in isolated units remote from the rest of their family, whose backgrounds and places of work he does not know, and who may have become his patients only in adult life, with their previous medical notes written in a totally indecipherable hand.

Sadly, the current trend toward holism within sections of the orthodox medical profession will not be easy to follow through; given today's larger and more mobile populations, we will never be able to return to the old family-doctor days. And no matter how holistically inclined a practitioner is, Western medicine per se is not a holistic therapy, since the majority of treatments now available involve the use of drugs or surgery. Surgery, of course, cannot be holistic—it is based on the principle that if a part of the patient is diseased, that part is removed. Drug therapy can be starkly contrasted with one of the complementary therapies, homeopathy. In order to work to the best advantage, a homeopathic remedy must relate to all aspects of the patient, not just to the symptoms of which he is complaining. Modern drugs, on the other hand, are formulated to have a specific action on only one or two particular complaints. So we have anti-arthritic drugs, hypotensive and cardioprotective drugs (to bring down the blood pressure and to protect the heart), tranquilizers and sleeping pills. And this is why people with several complaints find themselves having to take a number of different tablets to control them all. If a patient is suffering from bronchitis, arthritis, and bad eyesight, a holistic therapy used correctly may well produce an improvement in all three conditions, since its action is to raise the level of health of the whole patient, allowing his body to fight back against the problems that are troubling him. There is no way that a Western practitioner can prescribe a single medication that will do this, however, much as he might like to; nor has any orthodox drug been found that can raise a patient's entire level of health. The old-fashioned tonics were supposed to do this, although in fact they contained only stimulants such as strychnine, along with iron to cure any iron-deficiency anemia that might happen to be contributing to the patient's malaise. But this sort of treatment is quite possible for a truly holistic therapy.

The point about a holistic therapy is that it does not treat a single symptom, or even a disease. It treats a patient. And each patient is an individual unlike any other. Although they may not treat us as such, Western doctors are also well aware of this. The controlled trials that are used in Western medicine to compare two forms of treatment, or to establish the efficacy of a new treatment, involve using two comparable groups of patients. And it is not always easy to find enough "matched" patients, even when the matching criteria are as basic as age, sex, and the length of time that the patient has been ill. Think how much harder it would be to match patients if you also included things such as weight, temperament, marital status, number of children, job, level of education, financial status, housing, and so on. And yet all these things contribute to that patient being the person he is.

In a holistic therapy, then, every patient is treated individually, because what relieves the symptoms of one may have no effect at all on another who, in orthodox terms, appears to have the same complaint. Even in Western medicine it is acknowledged that patients react differently to different drugs. Not all patients with arthritis, for example, can be treated with the same medication; some will find it helpful, but others will show little response or will develop side effects whose severity outweighs the relief obtained from taking the drug. And this is one reason why a large number of drugs may be available for the treatment of a single condition. Most doctors have favorite drugs for common conditions—those that seem to them to be most effective and that they will always use as their first choice. But trying to find the right medication for a patient always has something of a hit-and-miss aspect to it, simply because a doctor can never tell in advance exactly how this patient, as opposed to the last patient or the next one, will respond to a particular drug.

In acupuncture, however, the system of diagnosis is geared to finding an individual tailor-made treatment for an individual patient. In Western medicine a diagnosis—and therefore the treatment of the patient of whom the diagnosis is made—is based on determining which particular organ, system, or part is malfunctioning. The diagnosis is made in terms relating to that part, such as *heart attack, gallbladder disease, kidney stones, slipped disk, varicose veins,* and so on. In other words, the diagnosis usually given is a description of the end result of the disease process. It is not related to any causative factors. This is not to say that Western medicine is not interested in preventive medicine, but the emphasis in disease remains firmly on the disease process and its end result.

Prevention, as well as diagnosis, can be undertaken on various levels. For instance, infection can be prevented in three ways. The first is to give the patient a prophylactic antibiotic so that, if his system is invaded by bacteria, the antibiotic will kill them and he will not become ill; the second is to examine the environment, find out where the bacteria are coming from, and eradicate them (this is the way in which most orthodox prevention works); the third way is to look at the patient and treat him as a whole, so that his own natural defenses are strong enough to resist any attack that may occur.

This third way is the holistic way—raising the patient's level of health—and is the basis on which patients are treated by acupuncture. The diagnosis is concerned with how the energies of the body are malfunctioning rather than with the manifestations of disease that a particular malfunction has caused. The area in which the disease appears (such as the heart, gallbladder, or kidney) is merely an indication of how the body has been affected by the disruption of its energies. In other words, heart disease does not mean that there is a problem heart in an otherwise healthy body, or even that the heart itself needs to be treated. What it does mean is that the patient's vital energies have become disrupted in a way that has manifested as disease of the heart. The disease manifestation is a clue to the acupuncturist as to how to treat the patient in order to restore him to health, but it is nothing more.

Here, then, is the basic difference between Western drug therapy and acupuncture. A patient who is prescribed drugs for his condition may be lucky the first time—many are—and rapidly obtain relief. Many others have to try a succession of possible treatments before they see any worthwhile improvement in their condition, however, and they may have to put up with unpleasant side effects along the way. But a patient being treated by an expert acupuncturist who makes a correct holistic diagnosis will be given a treatment that is tailored to his needs from the very beginning. Another major difference is that in many cases of chronic illness, such as arthritis, chronic bronchitis, or psoriasis, the patient who is treated by Western means may have to remain on medication for life, since the drugs, although possibly controlling the symptoms admirably, may have no effect on the underlying condition. Because acupuncture and other holistic therapies treat the body in such a way as to raise it to a level of energy at which it can heal itself, they may be able to reverse chronic diseases to a certain extent. After a successful course of treatment it may be months or even years before the patient needs to see his practitioner again.

It must be said, of course, that not every patient will respond to acupuncture, even in expert hands. Here again, the patient is an individual. In the same way that there is no one drug that suits every patient, there is no one therapy that suits everyone. Indeed, for those patients who respond well to Western therapy and experience no unpleasant side effects, there would seem to be no advantage in looking elsewhere, because sometimes people have to try more than one complementary therapy before finding the one that works for them.

CHI

The Chinese see the whole functioning of the body and mind as being dependent on the normal flow of body energies or life force, which they call Chi. In recent years a new way of interpreting Chinese words into Roman characters has been used and, nowadays, *Chi* is often spelled *Qi* or *Ki*. However, since in English the word is usually pronounced "chee," I prefer to retain the older spelling.

Chi, then, is the life force, but it is not just the life force of the individual person or animal, and my Chi is not distinct from your Chi. Chi is a universal energy that surrounds and pervades everything, both animate and inanimate. Like radio waves or ultraviolet light, we cannot see Chi or feel it. Like these other two energies, we can only recognize it in terms of what it effects. Radio waves, when picked up by a receiver tuned to the right frequency, will transmit sound. But a radio through which radio waves do not pass cannot itself produce any sounds. In the same way Chi is apparent to us as the life force of a body, and a body that no longer has Chi circulating through it is dead. But just as radio waves do not depend on radio sets for their existence and therefore do not disappear when a set is broken, so the Chi that permeates a body does not just disappear at its death. Chi is in a constant state of flux; there is constant interchange between the Chi of the body and Chi of the environment, or external Chi. And in the same way that food can be good or bad, nourishing or poisonous, external Chi can also be good or harmful.

Like air and food, Chi is taken in from the outside in the processes of breathing and eating. This external Chi is transformed within the body and used to replenish the internal Chi. Waste Chi is eliminated in the same way as the end products of respiration and digestion. Within the body Chi performs several specific functions, one of which is to form protective Chi. If this protective Chi is strong, it acts as a defense against any harmful external Chi with which you may come into contact. If your protective Chi is weak, however, then your resistance is lowered and you can be attacked by harmful external Chi. If this happens, the body becomes ill. This is a concept that is also understood, although in different terms, in Western medicine. Most people are aware that if they are run down or overtired, or if their diet is poor, they are more likely to suffer from infections. What a nutritionist would call vitamin-rich food might be referred to by a Chinese physician as food rich in Chi. This interesting analogy can, to a certain extent, be demonstrated physically by Kirlian electrography, a method in which an image is obtained on photographic paper of the energy (or corona discharge) emanating from a person or object. Its main use is as a diagnostic tool and an adjunct to complementary therapies, when pictures taken of a patient's hands and feet can point to abnormalities in the body's energy field. Pictures can also be obtained of inanimate objects. It has been found that foods high in nutritional value, such as green vegetables and whole-grain bread have a much better corona discharge than junk foods that contain few vitamins or minerals. Whether what the pictures show as a discharge is what the Chinese know as Chi has not yet been proved, but there is no doubt that when we eat nutritionally wholesome food, we are also ingesting some form of energy.

Thus the patient on a poor diet may be opening himself to attack by lowering his defenses. Stress, too, can break down our resistance to illness. Chinese medical theory recognizes that not all disease comes from outside as an attack by harmful Chi; it may also be due to imbalances arising within, often as a result of emotional problems.

Whether or not we get ill depends not just on the germs, carcinogens, and other outside influences waiting to attack us but also, and more importantly, on our own inner resistance or protective Chi. This idea is not alien to the thinking of Western physicians—although of course they express it in different terms. In his book *Cancer and Its Nutritional Therapies,* Dr. Richard A. Passwater writes that "fanatical avoidance of every possible carcinogen is not possible. They are everywhere. . . . The best hope remains in always retaining a strong immune response."

Whether we think in terms of Chi or of immune response, once we have become ill, our inner resistance is also of vital importance in determining how easily and quickly we get better. By raising our level of health, the therapist can reinforce our intrinsic resistance to disease, and thus we can be helped to heal ourselves.

Some people, of course, just never seem to get ill, whereas others are laid low by every bug that goes around. This is beautifully illustrated by a scene in Billy Wilder's film *The Apartment*. The hero, C. C. Baxter (played by Jack Lemmon), catches a streaming cold after he has been shut out of his apartment for the best part of the night in the pouring rain. The next morning he steps into the elevator at the New York insurance company where he works and tells the elevator operator (Shirley MacLaine) not to stand too close for fear of catching his germs.

"I never get colds," she says casually. C. C. Baxter is impressed. He tells her that he has been examining the statistics on colds and asks, "Did you know that the average New Yorker between twenty and fifty has two and a half colds a year?"

"That makes me feel just terrible," says the woman.

"Why?" asks Baxter.

"Well, to make the figures come out even, if I have no colds a year, some poor slob must have five colds a year."

"Yes," agrees Baxter, "it's me."

In Chinese terms people such as C. C. Baxter are out of balance, whereas Shirley MacLaine's elevator operator and others like her are in balance. If the woman had stayed out all night in the rain she probably wouldn't have caught a cold; at most she might have developed just a temporary sniffle. People such as this have strong protective Chi. They are taking in plenty of good Chi to replenish their internal Chi. And Chi is circulating around their bodies normally, not encountering any blockages and enjoying perfect balance between its opposing positive and negative aspects, yin and yang.

YIN AND YANG

Like Chi, yin and yang pervade everything. However, unlike Chi, they are not energies in themselves but rather aspects of everything, each being unable to exist without the other. You can think of them in the same terms as right and left: Neither can be described without reference to the other, and yet as a pair they are totally understandable and useful concepts. Yin and yang each have their own qualities and, because these qualities are the opposite of each other, yin and yang must be in perfect balance within the body in order to maintain perfect health. An imbalance will cause malfunction in the same way that an object that is much larger and heavier on its right side than on its left may well topple over.

Yin pertains to coldness, slowness, dimness, quietness, and solidity and is associated with female characteristics and the night. Yang, on the other hand, is hot, fast, bright, excited, and insubstantial, and is associated with the male characteristics and daytime. Anything that is interior, low down, or moving in a downward direction is yin. Anything that is exterior, high up, or moving upward is yang.

However, because there is a balance in everything, nothing is exclusively yin or exclusively yang—although it may be predominantly one or the other. There is something of both aspects in everybody and everything. Although a man is predominantly yang in his makeup, he has some balancing yin; similarly, a woman has a predominance of yin, but she still has a yang component.

Western medicine, too, recognizes that women have a male component and men a female component. The sex of a fetus is determined at conception: The fusion of an egg with a sperm carrying an X chromosome results in a girl, while fusion with a Y-carrying sperm produces a boy. In their early stages, however, all embryos develop in the same way, regardless of which sex they will ultimately be. The sexual organs develop from the same cells whether the baby is a boy or a girl, and it is at a fairly late stage of intrauterine development that physical differentiation takes place. At birth all babies are roughly the same shape, and with their diapers on it is often hard to tell boys from girls. The typical body shape and hair distribution of male and female develop in response to the hormones that are first secreted in large amounts at puberty. Because males can secrete some female hormones and females can secrete some male hormones, it is possible for women to become hairy or for men to develop breast tissue. This can sometimes occur in perfectly normal adolescents while their hormones are "sorting themselves out."

You could say that the hairy girl has a temporary excess of yang, while the boy whose breasts begin to swell has excessive yin. But the terms *yin* and *yang* encompass far more than just sexual characteristics. As components of all animate and inanimate objects, they are in a constant state of flux. According to how you look at something, its "yin-ness" and "yang-ness" change. For example, when you look at the body as a whole, the outside surface (being exterior) is yang and the inner organs (known as the zang-fu organs) are yin. But if you look only at the trunk, the back is primarily yang and the chest and abdomen (being the front, or the "inside" when you bend over) are yin. Then again, if you consider the chest and abdomen, the chest (being upper) can be said to be yang, and the abdomen (being lower) is yin. Thus yin and yang are not concrete characteristics of an object but are more relevant to that object's relationships to whatever is surrounding it. Here again, the comparison with the concepts of right and left is useful. If you describe your body, you will describe one arm as the left arm and the other as the right arm. However, you could also describe the inside border of your right arm as its left border, or the inside border of your left arm as its right border. So that which is right has an aspect of leftness, and vice versa. Similarly, because we always look at our own bodies from a looking-forward position, our right and left arms remain constant. But if we look at our environment, right and left are variable. Myrtle Street may be the first on the left past the church or the last on the right before the church, depending on where we are standing when we give the directions.

In all things that are opposite aspects of each other, there has to be balance, since by definition it is the two together that make the whole. You can't have right without left; nor can you recognize light without knowledge of darkness. And the balance that is essential within the body must also be maintained between the body and its environment.

In Western medical terms a fairly simple example of this can be given.

Sixty percent of the body is made up of water, and this water is distributed throughout the body. A certain amount of it is inside the body's cells; some makes up the interstitial fluids that flow around and between the cells, keeping them moist; the rest is in the body's fluids—the blood, lymph, saliva, digestive juices, and other secretions. It is very important that the amount of water in each section remains constant in relation to the others. The body would not be able to function if, when water was drunk, it flowed into a section haphazardly. For example, if excess water entered the bloodstream, the increased blood volume would cause the blood pressure to rise. Similarly, if too much water entered the tissue cells, this would cause edema (swelling of the tissues). Therefore the body has highly complex mechanisms by which the amount of water taken in is apportioned in the correct amounts to the various places where it is needed and so remains balanced.

Anything that has to keep a balance cannot be static or rigid, because it must always be ready to adapt to changes occurring around it. So the balance of yin and yang must always be fluid. It follows, therefore, that any condition that restricts this fluidity will affect the body's ability to maintain its own natural health. In Chinese terms many medical problems are associated with an imbalance of yin and yang, one or the other being either in excess or deficient. If yin becomes excessive, it will overwhelm the yang that is trying to balance it. This will result in a disease that has the characteristics of yin: coldness, slowness, and lack of activity. But the same type of disease can result if the excess of yin is only relative—in other words, if it is due to a deficiency of yang. In the same way, an excess of yang will overwhelm normal yin, producing a disease with yang characteristics—heat, excitement, and overactivity—which can also be a symptom of a lack of yin.

To a physician with Western medical training who is not looking at a patient in terms of yin and yang, someone with a deficiency of yang could appear to have an illness identical to that of another person who is suffering from an excess of yin. For example, such symptoms might be exhibited by a patient with myxedema, or thyroid deficiency, who would be treated with a thyroid supplement. However, if a patient with myxedema were seen by an acupuncturist, he might be diagnosed as having either an excess of yin *or* a deficiency of yang. And the acupuncturist would treat the patient with excessive yin differently from one with deficient yang, since he would try to bring back to normal the aspect that was malfunctioning.

The Chinese term for excess or fullness is *shi;* that for deficiency or emptiness is *xu*. Disease states in which the fundamental problem is one of excess (no matter what the excess) are thus known as shi syndromes, while those in which there is a deficiency of any sort are known as xu syndromes. A shi syndrome may be seen as one in which, although its natural resistance is intact, the body has been invaded and overwhelmed by an outside agent, while a xu syndrome is one in which the body's own defenses have been lowered to such an extent that it has no resistance. It is clear, therefore, why treatment of the two types of syndrome must differ from each other: in a xu syndrome it is necessary to reinforce the body's defenses against invasion (for example, deficient yin must be stimulated); in a shi syndrome, however, the treatment is to reduce the excessive factor.

A parallel can be found in Western medical terms. The white blood cells are the body's protection against infection. The production of these cells is dependent on a number of factors, not least on the dietary intake of certain essential nutrients such as vitamins C and E, zinc, and magnesium. If you get an infection, it may be either because your white blood cells are deficient or because the bacteria or viruses are too strong for your body's defenses. In the latter case (a shi syndrome) antibiotics would be needed to fight the bacteria, but in the former (a xu syndrome) it might only be necessary to supplement your diet to reinforce your natural defenses. (Many people do this by, for instance, taking large doses of vitamin C to treat a cold.)

A disruption in the balance between yin and yang, whether it is due to an excess or a deficiency, produces an abnormality in the flow of Chi in the affected area. When the balance of yin and yang is restored to normal, the flow of Chi will also return to normal.

CATEGORIES OF CHI

Chi itself can be divided into categories according to the function that it is performing. Having previously said that Chi is all-pervading and is in a constant state of flux, I realize that this may sound contradictory. However, a parallel with blood may make it clearer. The composition of one person's blood remains the same in terms of the number of red blood cells, white cells, and platelets in it, and in terms of the amount of iron in the red cells, no matter where in the body that blood is. However, other things about it will vary according to what its function is at the time. Arterial blood, which has just left the lungs, is carrying oxygen to the body tissues and will be bright red, while venous blood, which is returning to the lungs carrying carbon dioxide to be exhaled, is dark red. The portal vein carries blood containing the broken down products of protein, fats, and carbohydrates from the intestines to the liver, while blood entering the kidneys will contain waste products from body cells. But fundamentally, it is all the same blood; what is venous one minute can become arterial the next simply by passing through the lungs. Similarly, Chi can be divided into categories. Because it pervades everything, it is seen as being taken in with food and with the air you breathe. Inhaled air contains *clean Chi;* exhaled air contains *waste Chi.* These, together with the nutrients obtained from food, are known as *material Chi. Nourishing Chi* is derived from the digestion of food by the stomach and spleen and circulates through the meridians—which, like the arteries and veins that carry the blood, carry Chi around the body. It is these meridians that form the basis for acupuncture therapy. *Protective Chi,* which I have mentioned as being the body's natural defense against invasion, is also formed from food and circulates in the superficial tissues of the body and in the skin. Nourishing Chi is primarily yin, whereas protective Chi is primarily yang—again, two aspects of the same thing.

Each organ of the body has its own Chi, which is known as *functional Chi,* and it is this that maintains the normal function of that organ. However, all these different forms of Chi are interrelated and interdependent, in exactly the same way that venous blood becomes arterial after it has been through the lungs and arterial blood becomes venous after it has delivered its oxygen to the tissues. The purpose of protective Chi is to help defend the body from attack by harmful Chi, which can invade and cause illness. By stimulating and strengthening the level of protective Chi, acupuncture can be used as a preventive treatment.

THE MERIDIANS

Acupuncture treatment uses as its medium the meridians through which Chi flows. The meridians, like the blood vessels, have identical routes on the right and left sides of the body. In the same way that there is a right carotid artery and a left carotid artery, a right renal artery and a left renal artery, a right femoral vein and a left femoral vein, and so on, there are right and left Lung meridians, right and left Kidney meridians, and so forth. There is, however, a difference. If, for example, there is a malfunction of a vein on the left, in orthodox medicine it is the left vein only that will be treated, whereas in acupuncture treatment of either the left or right meridian of the pair will affect the other. Some authorities claim that to treat only the meridian opposite the one affected will produce an effect in 30 percent of cases; to treat only the affected meridian will produce an effect in 60 percent; and treatment of both together will produce an effect in 90 percent. Other practitioners, more cynical perhaps, say that the reason for this is that if you are inaccurate in locating the acupuncture points, then treatment of both sides gives an increased chance of actually hitting the right spot. Be this as it may, some practitioners always treat patients symmetrically. The fact that treatment of the opposite meridian will affect the disturbed meridian is very valuable when treating a patient in whom pain makes it impossible to treat the affected side. If someone is suffering from shingles, for example, the needles would commonly be put on the side of the body opposite the rash.

There are twelve pairs of meridians. Each half of a pair behaves exactly like its partner, unless one of them is diseased. It is easier, however, to speak of "the Lung meridian" than of "the two Lung meridians, left and right." This, therefore, is the terminology that is commonly used, and that I will use in this book.

In addition to the twelve major meridians, there are two that are unpaired, known as Du and Ren. They run down the midline of the body, back and front. There are also six other "extra" meridians made up of points from the major meridians that form links between them. The meridians are joined to each other by collaterals; these can be used to carry excess Chi from one that has too much to another that is deficient.

Each of the twelve major meridians is associated with an organ of the body—thus we have the Lung meridian, the Liver meridian, the Heart meridian, and so on. Each meridian receives Chi from another meridian and passes it on to a third, so that Chi circulates around the meridians in the same way that blood circulates through the blood vessels. In the latter case a number of factors can affect the amount of blood being carried by a vessel at any one time. For example, after a meal there will be an increased amount of blood in the vessels supplying the stomach and intestines; or when the weather is hot, there will be an increased blood supply to the skin so that heat can be radiated from the body (causing the flushed face characteristic of someone who is overheated). In contrast, the flow of Chi through the meridians is controlled by a strict biological clock.

Chi is said to surge in individual meridians at particular times. Each of the twelve major meridians is coupled with one of the others and, while Chi is surging in one of the couple, it will be at its lowest ebb in the other. So, for example, Chi is said to be at its maximum in the Liver meridian between 1 and 3 A.M., while its opposite number, the Small Intestine meridian, is at its lowest during this period. Between 1 and 3 P.M., however, the position is reversed, with the Small Intestine meridian having its maximum flow of Chi and the Liver meridian its lowest.

It has been suggested that jet lag may be due to the meridians not yet having adapted to the new time zone in which they have arrived. Going from London to New York, for instance, will find the Liver meridian having its maximum flow at around 8 in the evening instead of in the early hours of the morning, which is what it is used to. The symptoms of jet lag will persist until the meridians adapt to the new time zone.

The theory of the circulation of Chi is of use to the acupuncturist in both the diagnosis and the treatment of his patient. For example, a patient suffering from ulcerative colitis may often be woken by abdominal pain and a desire to have his bowels open at around 5 or 6 A.M. To the acupuncturist, the symptoms plus the timing suggest a disruption of Chi in the Large Intestine meridian, which has its maximum flow between 5 and 7 A.M. It is sometimes helpful, if possible, to treat a meridian during its period of maximum flow, and a patient may therefore be asked to make an appointment for a particular time of day. Obviously, this is more likely to be done with the meridians that have their surges of flow during the day than those that peak at night, since acupuncturists, like doctors, are unlikely to treat anything other than emergencies at night.

Each meridian is predominantly either yin or yang (although, of course, each will have aspects of both). In the coupling of meridians, each yin meridian is associated with a yang meridian so that when Chi is at its maximum in a yin meridian, it is at its lowest in a yang one and vice versa. The circulation of Chi around the meridians entails it passing through two yin meridians, followed by two yang meridians, then two yin meridians, and so on. Each yin meridian is associated with a so-called solid (or zang) organ, while yang meridians are associated with hollow (or fu) organs. This relates back to the association of yin with solidity and yang with lack of substance.

When looked at anatomically, not all the "solid" organs are truly solid, so it might be more appropriate to refer to them by the Chinese terms, *zang* and *fu*. The zang organs are the heart, the liver, the spleen, the lung, the kidney, and the pericardium (the fibrous sac that surrounds the heart and assists its contraction; in some Western books on acupuncture it is referred to as the heart constrictor). The fu organs are the small intestine, the large intestine, the stomach, the gallbladder, the urinary bladder, and the sanjiao. The latter is a Chinese concept and not an organ in its own right in Western terms. The word *sanjiao* may be translated as "three warmers." The term refers to the chest (or upper jiao), the upper abdomen (middle jiao), and the lower abdomen (lower jiao), which are related to each other by their function of warming the organs contained within them.

The routes taken by the meridians are also related to their yin or yang qualities. For example, yin meridians of the arm run down its inner aspect, while yang meridians run down the outside.

Each meridian is intimately related to the organ from which it gets its name. For example, the Lung meridian extends into the lung, the Liver meridian into the liver, and the Large Intestine meridian into the large bowel. The organs themselves can be affected by treatment of the corresponding meridian, and disorders of a particular meridian may manifest as symptoms associated with its organ. The diagrams on the following pages tell only half the story. They illustrate the part of the meridian that is used in treatment—in other words, the part that runs near the surface of the body and along which the acupuncture points lie. However, these surface meridians extend into internal meridians, which are the links between the acupuncture points (those sites into which needles are inserted during treatment) and the internal organs.

The Lung meridian, which is yin, runs superficially from just below the collarbone down the inside of the arm and into the thumb, where it ends next to the nail. This is shown in figure 1. When the meridians are listed,

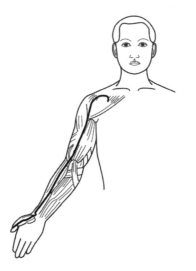

Figure 1. The Lung meridian

the Lung meridian is usually put first, since it is seen as being the starting point in the cycle of Chi. It has its surge of energy between 3 and 5 A.M., at which time its coupled meridian—that of the Urinary Bladder—is at its lowest. There are eleven acupuncture points lying along the course of the meridian; these are referred to either by their Chinese names or else as Lung 1, Lung 2 (often abbreviated Lu 1, Lu 2), and so on.

Interruption of the flow of Chi in the Lung meridian and consequent disruption of its function may be associated with chest symptoms such as cough, asthma, or tightness in the chest (associated with the internal course of the meridian and its link with the lungs), or with symptoms in the arm along the course of the superficial part of the meridian. When it affects a single meridian, either wholly or predominantly, the symptoms produced by an excess or a deficiency of Chi will be related to the function and course of that meridian and may be diagnostic. (More will be said about excess and deficiency syndromes in the next chapter.) An excess in the Lung meridian may produce a heavy feeling in the chest, shortness of breath, a severe cough with copious sputum, a dry and sore throat, a nasal discharge, redness of the bridge of the nose, and pain in the shoulder and arm. A deficiency may result in sneezing, a dry cough, dry skin, faintness, weight loss, shallow breathing, sensitivity to cold, and redness of the chin.

Figure 2 shows the Large Intestine meridian, which is the first of the two yang meridians that come immediately after the Lung meridian in the daily cycle of Chi. It surges between 5 and 7 A.M., when the Kidney meridian, with which it is coupled, is at its lowest. Because the Large Intestine meridian receives Chi directly from the Lung meridian, it begins very close to the end of the latter, its first point being next to the nail of the index finger. It is a yang meridian, so its course up the arm is along the outer aspect. Since it terminates so close to the nose, disruption of this meridian may be associated with nosebleeds. In addition, because it passes across the lower part of the face, it may be implicated in toothache. Sore throat and pain in the shoulder or arm are associated with the position of the rest of its superficial course. And because of its internal links with the large intestine itself, abdominal pain and diarrhea may also be symptoms

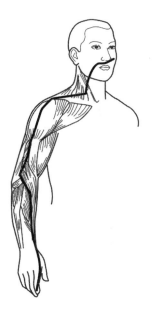

Figure 2. The Large Intestine meridian

of disruption of this meridian. An excess in the meridian is likely to cause pain along its course, stiffness of the shoulder, dizziness, abdominal distension, and constipation, while a deficiency may result in diarrhea, shivering, and a dry mouth. The Large Intestine meridian has twenty points along its superficial course, which are listed as LI 1, LI 2 . . . up to LI 20. In some books it is called the Colon meridian (*colon* being another name for the greater part of the large intestine), and in this case the abbreviation is Co 1, Co 2, and so on.

From the Large Intestine meridian Chi runs down the yang Stomach meridian, which is shown in figure 3 (page 46). Here again, the fact that it is a yang meridian is reflected in its course—which, when it runs down the leg, does so along the outer aspect. The Stomach meridian has its surge of Chi between 7 and 9 A.M., when the Pericardium meridian is at its lowest. Disruption of the flow of Chi in the Stomach meridian may produce symptoms associated with any part of its superficial course, such as nosebleed, sore throat, or chest pain. Symptoms related to the stomach itself, such as indigestion or upper abdominal pain, may also occur. An

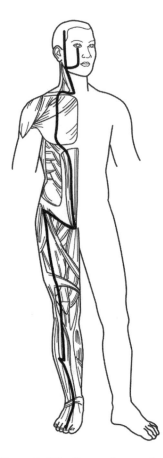

Figure 3. The Stomach meridian

excess in the meridian may cause an increase in appetite, constipation, thirst, bad breath, swelling and pain in the mouth, cramps in the legs, and fever. A deficiency may produce distension of the abdomen, diarrhea, vomiting, loss of appetite, and weakness in the legs. Forty-five points lie along the Stomach meridian, abbreviated St 1 to St 45.

The yin Spleen meridian continues the course of Chi, traveling from the big toe up the leg (along the inside, since it is a yin meridian) and over the abdomen to end a little way below the armpit. Its course is shown in figure 4. Interference with its function may cause vomiting, upper abdominal pain, jaundice, or diarrhea, all of which are related to its internal course

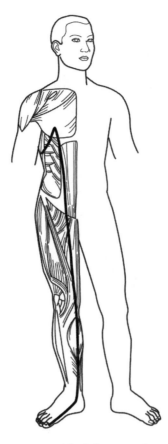

Figure 4. The Spleen meridian

and its path across the abdomen; or it may produce symptoms farther down in its course, such as painful or swollen knees. An excess affecting this meridian is likely to cause congestion in the chest with a productive cough, constipation, fatigue, and an irregular appetite. A deficiency may cause diarrhea and vomiting, flatulence, water retention, sleepiness, heaviness of the legs, and a poor memory. The Spleen meridian has twenty points, abbreviated Sp 1 to Sp 20, and its surge of Chi comes between 9 and 11 A.M., the Sanjiao meridian having the lowest flow at this time.

From the end of the Spleen meridian Chi is taken up by the yin Heart meridian, which runs from the armpit down the inside of the arm and

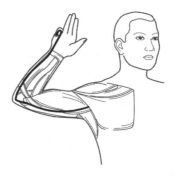

Figure 5. The Heart meridian

into the little finger, as shown in figure 5. Figure 6 shows how, from the little finger, it flows out again via the yang Small Intestine meridian up the outer (yang) aspect of the arm to just in front of the ear. The Heart meridian is one of the two shortest meridians, with only nine points along its course, abbreviated H 1 to H 9. Disruption of this meridian can cause symptoms that tie in well with the Western concept of heart disease, such as chest pain, palpitations, and pain in the arms, but because the heart in Chinese medicine is said to be the seat of the mind or spirit, it can also produce symptoms such as insomnia. An excess may be associated with a feeling of heaviness in the chest and a fever, while a deficiency may cause cold sweats, restlessness, palpitations, and a poor memory. The Chi in the Heart meridian (which is coupled with the Gall Bladder meridian) surges between 11 A.M. and 1 P.M.

Disruption of the Small Intestine meridian can produce deafness, sore throat, or pain in the shoulder and arm, all of which are related to its course; or abdominal pain, which is related to its inner links with the small bowel. Cold sores may be associated with an excess in this meridian, as may pain in the neck and shoulder. Ringing in the ears and a tender abdomen may be signs of a deficiency. Nineteen points lie along its course, shown as SI 1 to SI 19. Chi in the Small Intestine meridian surges between 1 and 3 P.M., when the flow in the Liver meridian is lowest.

Following on from the Small Intestine meridian, the yang Urinary Bladder meridian (sometimes referred to just as the Bladder meridian)

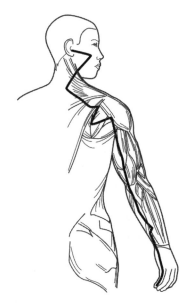

Figure 6. The Small Intestine meridian

takes Chi from the area between the eye and the nose up across the head, down through the neck, and along the side of the spine to the leg, where it travels down the back of the leg and into the foot to end in the little toe. Its route is shown in figure 7 (page 50). As you can see, the Urinary Bladder meridian also has an extra branch, which runs parallel to the first channel down the length of the spine.

Urinary problems are, naturally, associated with malfunction of this meridian. Pain anywhere along the length of the spine may also be a result of disruption of the flow of Chi in the Urinary Bladder meridian. Because the channel starts its external course just between the nose and the eye, injury to it may be responsible for nasal congestion, nosebleeds, headaches, watering eyes, and other eye problems. Frequent urination or bed-wetting may occur as a result of a deficiency in the meridian. I mentioned in connection with its paired meridian, that of the Lung, that the Urinary Bladder meridian is at its lowest ebb of energy between 3 and 5 A.M. This, of course, is a period of the night that is commonly associated with bed-wetting in children, and it is also the time at which many older people

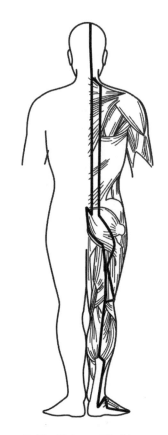

Figure 7. The Urinary Bladder meridian

find it necessary to get up in order to pass water. The surge of energy in the Urinary Bladder meridian comes at the opposite end of the day, between 3 and 5 in the afternoon. It is the longest of the meridians, mainly due to its parallel tracks down the vertebral column. There are sixty-seven points, which are commonly abbreviated UB 1 to UB 67 (Bl 1 to Bl 67 if it is being referred to simply as the Bladder meridian). However, the numbering of points along this meridian is not consistent in all books. Some authorities (usually Chinese) number the points starting at the eye and going down to the base of the spine (UB 1 to UB 35), then from below the buttock to the knee (UB 36 to UB 40), followed by the parallel course in the back (UB 41 to UB 54) and, finally, the section below the knee to the end of the meridian (UB 55 to UB 64). The other system of numbering, which seems to be favored in America, takes the sections in a different order so that after the first section (which remains the same) the parallel course in the back becomes UB 36 to UB 49; the final section goes from below the buttock to the foot and is numbered UB 50 to UB 67.

Next in the cycle is the yin Kidney meridian, which is shown in figure 8. It begins, as you might guess, near the termination of the Urinary Bladder meridian, in the foot. Beginning on the sole, it runs up the leg (along the inside, since it is a yin channel) and then up the abdomen, near the midline, to finish just below the inner aspect of the collarbone. It has its surge of energy between 5 and 7 P.M., and the twenty-seven points that lie along its course are abbreviated to K 1 to K 27.

Urinary problems may also be associated with abnormalities in the

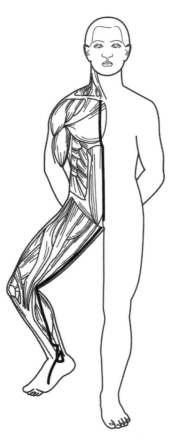

Figure 8. The Kidney meridian

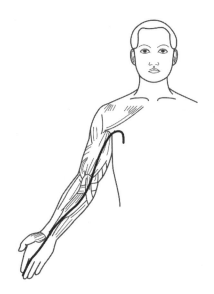

Figure 9. The Pericardium meridian

Kidney meridian. However, unlike the Urinary Bladder meridian, that of the Kidney also regulates sexual function, so disruption of its flow of Chi may cause menstrual problems in women or impotence in men. Its course across the chest means that asthma, coughing of blood, and sore throat may all be associated with problems in the Kidney meridian, and its course down the leg may produce local pain as a symptom of malfunction. An excess in the meridian may cause the patient to become hyperactive, while a deficiency can produce a loss of sex drive and a general timidity; both may be associated with ringing in the ears (more will be said about the kidney's link with the ears later on).

Following on from the Kidney meridian is the yin Pericardium meridian, which is illustrated in figure 9. The yang Sanjiao meridian, shown in figure 10, then carries Chi from the ring finger up the arm (the outer aspect, since it is a yang meridian) into the shoulder, up the side of the neck, around the ear, to finish next to the outer end of the eyebrow. The Pericardium meridian, like that of the Heart with which it is closely associated, has only nine points, listed as P 1 to P 9—or in some books as HC 1 to HC 9, where *HC* stands for Heart Constrictor. The Sanjiao meridian also has

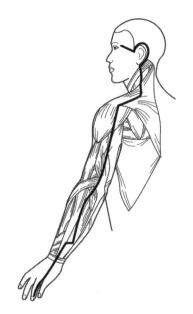

Figure 10. The Sanjiao meridian

two English names, with its twenty-three points listed either as SJ 1 to SJ 23 or as TH 1 to TH 23, *TH* being the abbreviation for Triple Heater. Chi surges through the Pericardium meridian between 7 and 9 P.M. and through the Sanjiao meridian between 9 and 11 P.M.

It can be seen from figure 9 that the course of the Pericardium meridian runs more or less parallel to that of the Heart meridian. Since the pericardium surrounds the heart, its meridian is associated with heart problems, including chest pain, palpitations, and shortness of breath. Malfunction of the Pericardium meridian can also produce anxiety and mental disturbance (because the heart is the seat of the mind). Headache, abdominal pain, and fever may be associated with an excess affecting the Pericardium meridian, while a deficiency can cause palpitations, shortness of breath, indigestion, and diarrhea; restless sleep may result from either. Disruption of the Sanjiao meridian can cause problems associated with any of the three cavities. For example, abdominal pain or distension may relate to the middle cavity, or jiao, and pain on passing urine to the lower jiao. But symptoms may also be related simply to its course. These include ringing in the ears, sore throat, and pain in the shoulders or arms. Such pain may relate to an excess in the meridian, as may sore throat, hearing difficulties, constipation, and retention of urine. A deficiency may be associated with nervousness and restlessness, diarrhea, incontinence, or water retention.

The yang Gall Bladder meridian, whose energy surges between 11 P.M. and 1 A.M., follows on from the Sanjiao meridian. Its long and somewhat convoluted route is shown in figure 11. Here again, as a yang meridian it runs down the outside of the leg. Disruption of the flow of Chi may cause symptoms related to any part of its superficial course, such as headache, blurring of vision, or pain in the chest, upper abdomen, or legs. An excess

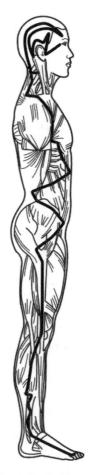

Figure 11. The Gall Bladder meridian

in the meridian may produce an increased appetite, abdominal pain, or jaundice, while a deficiency may be responsible for dizziness, anxiety, and insomnia. Forty-four points, GB 1 to GB 44, lie along its course.

The Liver meridian is a yin meridian and runs, as you can see in figure 12, from the big toe up the inside of the leg to the trunk, where it ends just below the nipple. This meridian is at its highest point of energy between 1 and 3 in the morning. Disruption of its function may be associated with pain anywhere along its superficial course, but particularly in the lower abdomen and upon passing water. Its course passes through the groin, and therefore hernias may be associated with its malfunction. So too may a feeling of tightness in the lower part of the chest and hiccups (which are

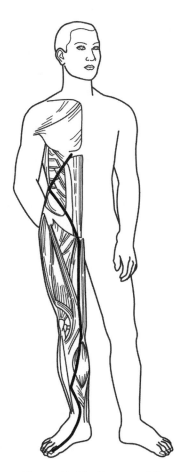

Figure 12. The Liver meridian

due to spasmodic contractions of the diaphragm—a large sheet of muscle that is attached to the lower border of the ribs and separates the abdomen from the chest). The liver is said to have specific functions, which I will describe in the next chapter. These are not the same functions as those accorded to it in Western medicine, and they may be disrupted by malfunction of the Liver meridian, producing symptoms such as headache and mental disturbance. An excess in the meridian may be associated with an unstable temperament, hyperactivity, and abdominal pain, while a deficiency may cause dizziness, poor eyesight, and dry skin. The Liver meridian has fourteen points, usually abbreviated Liv 1 to Liv 14 but shown as Li in some books.

From the Liver meridian, the circulation of Chi is completed by the Lung meridian, which takes it up again from under the collarbone.

The total number of points on these twelve meridians is 309—although of course this is the number of points on just one side of the body. Since each of the meridians is bilateral, there are 618 points available for use. The Du meridian (sometimes called the Governing Vessel and abbreviated GV), disruption of which may be associated with back pain and headache, contributes a further twenty-eight points. It runs up the midline of the body from the base of the spine over the head to the center of the top lip. It forms a circle with the Ren meridian, also known as the Vessel of Conception and abbreviated VC, or sometimes CV. Abnormalities in this meridian are associated with menstrual problems, vaginal discharge, retention of urine, and abdominal pain. The Ren meridian has twenty-four points along its course, which runs from the center of the perineum (the area between the legs, in front of the anus) up the midline of the abdomen and chest, to finish just below the center of the lower lip. The course of these two meridians is shown in figures 13 and 14.

There are also extra meridians that link points from the other main meridians. For example, the Yangwei meridian (a yang meridian, naturally) runs through points on the yang Urinary Bladder, Gall Bladder, Small Intestine, Sanjiao, Stomach, and Du meridians, while the Yingwei meridian (a yin meridian) joins points on the yin Kidney, Spleen, Liver, and Ren

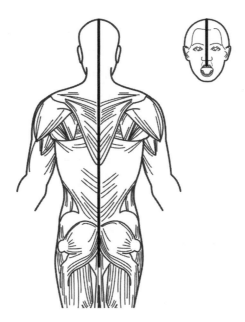

Figure 13. The Du meridian (Governing Vessel)

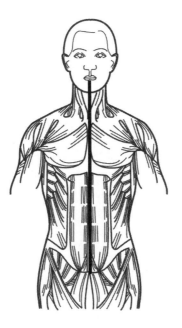

Figure 14. The Ren meridian (Conception Vessel)

meridians. The Du meridian is yang since it runs down the back, or outside, of the body; the Ren meridian, running down the inside, is yin.

Finally, there are also twenty extra points that are not connected with any specific meridian. Since Chi must, by its nature, circulate through the entire body, an acupuncture point does not necessarily have to be on a meridian, in the same way that you do not have to cut through a vein or artery in order to bleed.

The total number of acupuncture points from the twelve meridians, the two midline meridians, and the extra points is thus 381: 309 plus 28 plus 24 plus 20. (Modern researchers have discovered a large number of extra points, though 381 is still considered the basic figure.) It is interesting to note that the *Nei Ching* refers to 365 points, demonstrating that very little has changed in the basic theory of acupuncture in two thousand years.

3

The Five Elements

Each of the twelve major meridians is related to one of the elements recognized in classical Chinese philosophy—earth, wood, water, metal, and fire. These elements are understood to be intimately associated with all things, including the human body. Four meridians are associated with fire, while the other elements are associated with two meridians each. In some cases the reasoning behind the association is obvious (for example, the Urinary Bladder and Kidney meridians are linked to water); in others it is understandable (such as the linkage of the Heart meridian with fire). In addition to the overall association, each meridian has five acupuncture points that are related to each of the five elements.

One of the fundamentals of holistic practice is that no one part of the body can be disrupted in any way, no matter how small, without it having an effect on other parts. Figure 15 (page 61) shows how the meridians and their associated elements are related to each other according to the Law of the Five Elements. Disruption of the flow of Chi in one meridian is likely, directly or indirectly, to affect others. This means that the meridian in which the patient's symptoms are apparent is not necessarily the meridian that needs treating. The underlying cause may be in another meridian, whose disruption has caused abnormalities to occur in the symptom-producing meridian.

The rules that govern the effects of elements on each other, and therefore of meridians on each other, are known as the mother-child rule and the servant-master rule. It is said that in the same way that a mother gives birth to a child and nourishes him, so elements promote and nourish other elements. Wood is said to promote fire because it is combustible; a log fire that is deprived of wood to burn will go out. Fire in turn promotes earth by creating ashes. Even nowadays certain forms of ash are used as fertilizers to nourish the earth. Earth promotes metal because metal is dug out of the earth and so is engendered by it. Metal promotes water—with a stretch of the imagination—by melting, and water promotes wood by nourishing the tree, for a tree that is deprived of water will die.

By analogy, then, when a meridian associated with Wood (the Liver or the Gall Bladder meridian) is functioning normally, it will promote the normal flow of Chi and normal function in the Fire meridians (Heart, Pericardium, Small Intestine, and Sanjiao). In turn the normal function of the Fire meridians promotes flow in the Earth meridians (Spleen and Stomach), which, in the same way, nourish the Metal meridians (Lung and Large Intestine). These promote the function of the Water meridians (Urinary Bladder and Kidney), which complete the circle by nourishing the Wood meridians.

It follows that disruption in the flow of Chi in one meridian can disrupt flow in the meridian that it normally promotes or nourishes. If the disruption is allowed to continue untreated, it may go a step farther, affecting the meridian that is nourished by the second meridian involved. In this way the condition can spread to involve the entire body and meridian system.

The servant-master rule produces a different cycle of events. It is said that just as a master gives orders to his servant and controls his actions, so elements affect others by maintaining control over them. It is this control by the master, as much as the nourishment obtained from the mother, that enables the element in question to function normally. Wood is said to control earth, since trees grow on it and over it. Earth, in turn, controls water by damming it and so forcing it to flow in certain directions. Water controls fire, naturally enough, by extinguishing it, and fire controls metal by melting it. Metal controls wood by being made into tools that can cut it and fashion it into other things, and this completes the circle. So the Wood meridians (Liver and Gall Bladder) exert control over the Earth meridians (Spleen and Stomach). These two then control the Water meridians (Urinary Bladder and Kidney), which control the Fire meridians (Small Intestine, Sanjiao, Heart, and Pericardium). The Fire meridians control the Metal meridians (Lung and Large Intestine), and the latter control the Wood meridians. A malfunction in a meridian may be produced by a malfunction in which the master meridian exerts either inadequate or excessive control over its servant. In the latter case the Chi of the servant meridian may be reduced or—if the servant "rebels" against the increased control—may be excessive.

According to the Law of the Five Elements, each meridian has four connections. It is nourished by one meridian and controlled by another. It nourishes a third and controls a fourth. So each element is connected with every other element, as figure 15 shows, either as a mother, a child, a

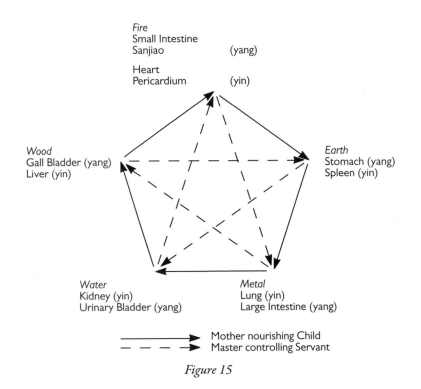

Figure 15

master, or a servant. In this respect the yin meridians primarily affect and are affected by the other yin meridians, and the yang meridians primarily affect and are affected by the other yang meridians.

It may be helpful here to look at one meridian and see how it can be affected by other meridians according to the mother-child and the servant-master rules. If we take as our example the Heart meridian—a yin Fire meridian—we will see that it is nourished by its mother, the yin Wood meridian, and in turn nourishes its child, the yin Earth meridian. It is controlled by its master, the yin Water meridian, and exerts control over its servant, the yin Metal meridian. This means that the Heart meridian is nourished by the Liver meridian while giving nourishment to the Spleen meridian, and is controlled by the Kidney meridian while controlling the Lung meridian.

It follows from this that a malfunction of the Heart meridian may be intimately related to a malfunction of the Liver, Spleen, Kidney, or Lung meridians. If the disorder originated in one of the other meridians, then treatment of the Heart meridian alone will not resolve the problem. The whole system must be balanced before the body can become healthy again.

I have heard a Western medical practitioner say that he thought acupuncture must be an easy therapy to master—"you just learn what each point does and then stick in your needles." But what I have just said about the Law of the Five Elements should make it clear that this is not the case. Acupuncture is not about diseases but about energy flow. And therefore it is not a case of learning that "this point cures headache and that one will stop vomiting." Each point has a specific function, sure enough, but this function has to do with moving energies. And so before a practitioner can use the points correctly, he must learn not only what each point does but also how to make a diagnosis in terms of what has gone wrong with the energy flow. Admittedly, there are some points with specific actions, such as the control of vomiting, but to use points only for this type of action without any knowledge of the theory of the flow of Chi is to use acupuncture at a fairly primitive level. The difference, perhaps, is similar to that between someone with a first-aid certificate and a surgeon. The former may certainly be useful in an emergency, but you would not expect him to produce the same results as the surgeon. Indeed, if the first-aider tried to ape the surgeon's work, he might end up doing more harm than good. To learn the basic theory of acupuncture in order to use it fully, correctly, and in a truly holistic way takes at least three years. The skill of the acupuncturist lies in diagnosing where the imbalance of Chi lies. In order to do this he has to know all the laws governing the behavior of the meridians and of the Chi flowing in them. I will say more about diagnosis in the next chapter.

Let us return now to the Heart meridian—which, as you have seen, is closely related through the Law of the Five Elements to the Liver, Spleen, Kidney, and Lung meridians. According to this law, a deficiency of Chi in its mother Liver meridian could cause the Heart meridian to become undernourished so that it, too, would develop a deficiency of Chi. Similarly, an excess of Chi in the Liver meridian could spill over and cause Chi in the Heart meridian to become excessive. A deficiency originating in the Heart meridian itself would deprive its child, the Spleen meridian. A condition in which the symptoms appear to be related to one meridian but are in fact due to a deficiency in the mother meridian is known as the screaming child syndrome—and the child will go on screaming until it is nourished.

A deficiency in the Heart meridian could also track backward in the cycle and produce a deficiency in the Liver meridian by "sucking it dry." An excess of Chi can also be transmitted either way, from mother to child or from child to mother. If a deficiency or an excess is found in the Liver, Heart, and Spleen meridians, this may well have originated from a primary disorder of the Heart meridian. In such a case treatment of the Heart meridian alone may resolve the problem.

The liver itself, as distinct from its meridian, is said by Chinese physicians to store blood and control the volume of the circulating blood. But the function of the liver is dependent on the normality of its related meridian. If there is a deficiency of Chi in the Liver meridian, not only Chi but also blood may be deficient. This would have an effect on its child, the Heart meridian, and on its child's related organ, the heart.

Western medicine also recognizes a link between the liver and the heart, although it is not expressed in the same terms as in Chinese medicine. The liver is the storehouse for various vitamins and minerals, including iron and vitamin B_{12}, which are essential for normal blood formation. A deficiency in the liver in Western terms (that is, a depletion of its nutritional stores) may have a serious effect on the blood, causing anemia. If severe enough, this may put stress on the heart and affect its action.

Another intimate relationship acknowledged by Western medicine is between the spleen and the heart—in Chinese terms the child and its mother. Red blood cells, which are responsible for carrying oxygen in the blood, have a life span of about 120 days. As cells reach this age, they are broken down by the spleen, and the iron that is released from them is reused by the bone marrow to produce new red blood cells. There are some forms of anemia—known as hemolytic anemias—in which excessive quantities of red blood cells, young as well as old, are broken down. This may put the heart under strain. Indeed, a sudden and overwhelming hemolytic crisis may precipitate heart failure. Although Chinese medicine does not describe the physiological function of the spleen in breaking down old red blood cells, it says that the spleen is the organ responsible for controlling the blood inside the blood vessels and preventing it from leaking out.

As we have seen, good health entails a normal balance between the body energies and the Chi of all the meridians. If a meridian fails, it may lose its control over its servant meridian. In this way a failing Kidney meridian can lose control over its servant, the Heart meridian, or a failing Heart meridian (in the role of master) can lose control over the Lung meridian. A similar sort of relationship whereby one system is controlled by another is understood in Western medicine. For example, a hormone is produced by the pituitary gland that stimulates the thyroid gland to produce hormones of its own. High levels of circulating thyroid hormones should cause the pituitary to switch off its hormone secretion, whereas low levels should stimulate it—but this biofeedback mechanism can break down.

A patient with an overactive or underactive thyroid gland may therefore have a problem either in the gland itself or in the pituitary—which has, so to speak, lost control.

The servant-master relationship is therefore one in which overactivity or underactivity of a meridian or its related organ may be associated with a loss of control or an excess of control by the master meridian. The Kidney meridian controls the Heart meridian, and the Heart meridian controls the Lung meridian. These three organs, the kidney, heart, and lung, are also recognized as being intimately related by Western physicians. The function of the kidneys is to maintain a balance of water and of minerals within the body. They also eliminate waste products, drugs, and other toxins from the body by filtering the blood to remove waste, toxins, water, and minerals, and then returning to the clean blood exactly the right amounts of water and minerals to keep the body in balance. The waste matter, rejected matter, and excess water are excreted as urine. If the kidneys fail to function normally, there is a buildup of toxins in the body, as well as retention of water and excessive minerals. The result is a rise in blood pressure. This affects the heart (whose meridian, according to Chinese theory, is controlled by that of the kidney). A continually raised blood pressure may finally result in heart failure, and this in turn causes fluid to accumulate in the lungs. In the West this would be called pulmonary edema, but looked at through an acupuncturist's eyes, it might be seen as a case of the heart failing to control the lungs. As we shall see in the next chapter, the lung is one of the organs said by the Chinese to be responsible for the normal distribution of water around the body.

These relationships have been expressed here in rather simplistic terms; in both Western and Chinese medicine the picture is somewhat more complicated. However, it does help to illustrate that in both systems the functions of these organs are interrelated.

The meridians that relate to each other as mother-child and servant-master are linked by specific points, the needling of which can open a channel between the two in order to allow Chi to flow from one to the other and so return to a state of equilibrium. Various points are available on each meridian by which transfer of Chi can be effected, and every meridian has a point relating to each of the elements: earth, water, fire, metal, and wood. These points are all to be found on the distal parts of the limbs. On the meridians that run through the arms, the points are around and below the elbow; on those that run through the legs, they are around and below the knee. It is these points that may be used to transfer Chi to and from the meridian associated with each element. Other points also have specific functions in terms of the transfer of Chi and particular effects on the meridian in question. These will be mentioned later.

Over the thousands of years that acupuncture has been used in China, two major systems of diagnosis and treatment have developed. One is based entirely on the Law of the Five Elements. The other, while using this law, also diagnoses according to the Eight Principles (sometimes called the Eight Conditions or Eight Syndromes), which I will describe in the next chapter. The fact that there are two systems does not mean that one is wrong and the other right, or even that one is superior to the other. In acupuncture, the diagnosis is more a means to an end than a concrete entity. It is a signpost, indicating to the practitioner which points he should use in order to restore balance to the patient's body energies. Both systems work to restore balance and both are effective in this respect. That they achieve their results by working from different angles is not important.

In this book I am going to concentrate mainly on diagnosis and treatment according to the Eight Principles, since this is the system with which I am more familiar. However, in chapter 7 I quote case histories from both traditions, so before explaining the Eight Principles I shall give a brief outline of the diagnosis used in the Five Elements system.

When a practitioner of the Five Elements system makes a diagnosis, he does so according to the element that is disturbed. A patient is seen as having a susceptibility to injury of a particular element that may stem from trauma in childhood or even from when he was still in the womb. Further trauma later in life is therefore likely to affect the meridians related to that element. Once this has occurred, the disturbance may spread to other meridians according to the mother-child and servant-master connections.

The practitioner will treat his patient with the aim of restoring balance among the meridians by removing excess Chi or stimulating a deficiency of Chi. His diagnosis is based on a number of factors such as the patient's color, his voice, his emotions, and his body odor.

A patient with a disturbance of the wood element is likely to have a greenish look to his skin, a rancid odor, and a loud aggressive voice. He may be irritable, restless, and unstable, and may be subject to depression.

If the fire element is affected, the patient will have a red face, a scorched body odor, and a normal or laughing quality of voice. He may have very labile emotions, being up one minute and down the next.

The earth patient has a yellowish look, a fragrant body odor, and a singing quality to his voice. He may be obsessional, tense, and overanxious, and may have a craving for sympathy.

A patient whose Metal meridians are affected will have a white complexion, a rotten smell, and a weeping quality of voice. He is likely to relate his story in grief-laden tones and to regard his problems with a great deal of negativity.

Finally, the water patient has a bluish look, a putrid smell, and a groaning voice. He is likely to be timid and fearful.

These, of course, are just the bare bones on which the practitioner bases his diagnosis. Among other things, he will also use pulse diagnosis (which I shall describe in chapter 5) to confirm which meridians are affected and in which way they are malfunctioning—that is, whether there is an excess or a deficiency. He may then use a variety of points to stimulate or sedate a meridian or to transfer energy from one element to another.

4

Causes of Disease

As we have seen, one of the causes of disease, according to traditional Chinese thinking, is invasion by harmful Chi. We may think of this invasion and the consequent effect that it has on the body in rather the same terms as the Western concept of infection and immunity. If the patient's protective Chi is at a low level, harmful Chi is able to invade and may overwhelm him because his body is unable to fight back. This is similar to the patient whose immune system is not working at full strength because he is taking massive doses of steroids after a transplant operation, or because he has an abnormality of his blood such as leukemia, or, on a less dramatic scale, because he is overtired or has a poor diet. Any of these will lower his resistance to some extent and make him susceptible to infection.

Exceptionally strong harmful Chi can also invade even if the body's protective Chi is normal. This may be compared with a particularly virulent infection that attacks healthy people whose immune systems are unimpaired. Invasion by harmful Chi in this instance may initially cause illness but, as long as the invading force is not too strong, the fact that the protective Chi is normal may allow the body to muster its forces and fight back (as indeed it does in many self-limiting infections). Long-term, chronic illness may be due to a balance developing between harmful Chi and protective Chi so that while the former is not overwhelming, it is too strong for the protective Chi to fight off entirely.

Disease is not always classified by the Chinese as coming from outside the patient. It can also be caused from within and, in this case, may be due to emotional upset, inherited factors, or a faulty diet. In the system of acupuncture based on the Eight Principles there are said to be seventeen major causes of disease: the six external factors, the seven emotional factors, and the four miscellaneous factors. In addition to these, disease can be due to trauma, poisoning, or other physical factors.

It is in terms of these causes of disease that the acupuncturist makes his diagnosis. Unlike a Western physician, who will diagnose in terms of which part of the body is diseased and what the abnormality is (for example, inflammation of the appendix, cancer of the lung, cysts in the ovaries, and so on), the acupuncturist will make his diagnosis according to what has caused the illness and what effect it has had on the body's energies and the function of the zang-fu organs. In this chapter I shall explain the effects said to be produced by the seventeen different causative factors.

THE SIX EXTERNAL FACTORS

The six external factors—wind, cold, damp, dryness, heat, and summer (or damp) heat—are all forms of harmful Chi. Of course, because this form of diagnosis developed in China, these factors originally related to the specific weather conditions prevailing in that part of the world. However, the fact that these were derived in a different climate from our own does not mean that they are invalid in the West, although the frequency of any one type of weather may differ from place to place. Londoners, for example, might be expected to have more illness related to dampness than, say, New Yorkers—who on the other hand might expect more illness of the summer heat type.

When the Chinese talk about invasion by an external factor, what they mean is an invasion by the essential characteristics of that factor, resulting in a disease that reflects those characteristics. In other words, you would not expect a patient who has been invaded by cold necessarily to have a lower temperature than normal; nor does invasion by wind necessarily cause flatulence!

WIND

Wind is said to be prevalent in the spring although, in the West, it is perhaps somewhat more common in the autumn. People are said to be more susceptible to wind diseases if they are exposed to this element when they are hot or have been sweating profusely, or if they have been sleeping in a draft. Wind is predominantly yang, reflecting this in its attributes—it is always moving, insubstantial, and agitated, and is often said to attack the upper (yang) part of the body. Wind is thought to enter the body through the pores of the skin, disrupting their functioning so that the patient may sweat excessively. Headache is also a common symptom of diseases caused by wind.

The patient is not always attacked by wind from outside, for it can also develop from within the body as a result of an excess of yang arising in the liver. The symptoms of internally created wind diseases differ somewhat from those produced by external wind. In the first case the complaint might be of ringing in the ears and muscle spasms, together with dizziness and headache. In the latter the dizziness and headache might be associated with sore throat and a raised temperature.

As I noted, the symptoms of the diseases caused by the external factors usually have the characteristics of those factors. Diseases caused by wind thus tend to have symptoms that, like wind, are constantly changing or moving. A typical case would be a patient with rheumatic fever. Classically, the patient complains of joint pains lasting perhaps no more than a day before they move to another site; this is combined with fever and sweating. The sweating, as I have mentioned, is related to the wind's effect on the pores of the skin, while the fever relates to the yang qualities of wind, since yang is associated with heat. The patient may also have the headache characteristic of wind-induced diseases, and—particularly if the disease has been caused by external wind—he may have a dislike of being in a windy place.

Convulsions, spasms, and twitches of all types are said to be due to wind, as is facial paralysis, which causes a distortion of the features. This latter seems reminiscent of the English folklore cited by mothers who, to stop their children from making faces, tell them, "If the wind changes, you'll get stuck like that."

COLD

The external factor of cold is, of course, prevalent in the winter and is more likely to attack someone if he is not warmly dressed or is exposed to the cold after getting overheated. Cold is a yin characteristic so, when it invades, it overwhelms the body's yang Chi, resulting in an imbalance between yin and yang.

The symptoms of disease caused by cold are those you might expect with an excess of yin—coldness, slowness, and inhibition of function. The patient may complain of feeling cold and may shiver and look pale. His feet and hands may be numb or go blue due to poor circulation, and he may have cramps in his muscles. Usually these symptoms are associated with a dislike of the cold. Invasion by cold of the internal organs, particularly of the intestines, may cause diarrhea and abdominal pain. Cold is also associated with stiffness and stagnation—a sort of "icing up" of the body. The blood and Chi are both liable to stagnate in the presence of cold, and the resulting accumulation of either may cause localized pain. So arthritis, in which the patient experiences stiffness and localized areas of pain, may be due to cold. In such cases the patient may well find that his condition deteriorates during cold weather.

An attack of flu in which the patient shivers and complains of aching muscles may also be ascribed to invasion by cold. There may be fever in cold diseases, but it is not accompanied by excessive sweating. Frostbite is one condition in which Western medical diagnosis would agree with traditional Chinese medicine that the symptoms—numbness in the feet and hands associated with pallor or blueness—are due to invasion of the body by cold.

Like wind, cold may arise internally. With its yin characteristics, it can develop as a result of a weakness in the yang of the body, which thus becomes overwhelmed by yin. A patient who has a cold disease that has arisen internally is more susceptible to external cold than a healthy person, since he has inadequate yang with which to resist it. If he is invaded by external cold, this will exacerbate his condition and may precipitate a crisis.

DAMP

Damp in China was said to cause problems mainly in the late-summer rainy season. In Japan, as I noted in chapter 1, it is a far more frequent cause of illness, occurring all year round. Damp-induced diseases are said to be caused by wearing wet clothes for any length of time or by constantly being in a damp environ-ment. Damp is described as heavy and stagnant in character, and the diseases that are caused by it have similar characteristics, tending to be long-term problems. The symptoms may include a heavy feeling in the body and the head; the patient may suffer from dizziness. Swelling of the abdomen or ankles (known, in Western terms, as fluid retention) may occur, and the nose and chest may feel stuffy. Heaviness and chronicity are yin characteristics, and therefore damp is predominantly yin. If dampness arises from within, it attacks the yang of the spleen and damages it. This can cause chronic digestive problems (since the spleen is considered to be an important digestive organ), and the patient may suffer from recurrent attacks of watery stools or diarrhea.

Damp causes stagnation and, in the same way that stagnant water is often polluted and foul smelling, damp is said to cause foul discharges. Foul-smelling and profuse vaginal discharges, smelly infected urine, and oozing skin conditions are all damp associated.

When damp attacks the upper part of the body, it produces a heavy feeling in the head, a blocked nose, yellowness of the face, and difficulty in breathing. These symptoms are not unlike those that might appear, according to Western diagnosis, in a patient suffering from Weil's disease—which, interestingly enough, is an infection spread by rats living in or near stagnant water, and which is an occupational hazard for sewage workers.

DRYNESS

In China diseases caused by dryness are associated with the late autumn—a time that in Europe and the United States is more likely to be associated with damp and wind. Dryness, of course, is said to affect the body's fluids. In Chinese medicine, as in Western, it is recognized as essential that the body fluids be kept in balance. This balance, in Chinese thinking, is intimately associated with the balance of yin and yang. Dryness itself is primarily yang and therefore can be especially destructive to yin fluid, particularly that of the lung, causing a dry cough associated with a sore throat and dryness of the mouth and nose.

Dryness may be subdivided into cold dryness and warm dryness. The symptoms of cough and dryness of the throat are common to both, but a patient affected by cold dryness may also have a headache and a dislike of the cold, while a patient whose symptoms are due to warm dryness may be feverish and sweaty.

As you might expect, all dry-skin conditions, such as certain types of dermatitis, are said to be due to dryness. So too are wasting diseases in which the patient looks as though he has been literally dried out, like a prune. Tuberculosis, when it affects the lung, has the characteristics of dryness, being associated with a dry chesty cough and a general wasting of the body.

Since dryness is yang associated, it may develop internally as a result of yin deficiency. However, it may also occur if bodily fluids are lost through diarrhea, vomiting, or excessive sweating, and may thus complicate another disease process.

HEAT AND SUMMER (OR DAMP) HEAT

Heat, which is yang in character, overwhelms the body's yin Chi when it invades and upsets the natural balance of yin and yang. Summer heat is regarded as different from heat itself, Chinese summer heat being heavy and damp. Despite the damp element, the yang component is strong, and so yang symptoms are still produced. The person who tends to be affected by summer heat is one who remains out in the hot sun for a long time or stays in a room with poor ventilation on a very hot day—the kinds of factors that are known by Western doctors to lead to heatstroke.

Summer heat overwhelms the body's yin and injures the body's fluids. It may also affect the mind, causing delirium or coma. Because heat is yang, and because yang is associated with acute onsets, the disease may start suddenly. Other symptoms of summer heat include profuse sweating and thirst with a fever and restlessness—all yang characteristics. Heatstroke, as defined in Western terms, shows all these attributes—thirst, fever, and restlessness—and may also affect the patient's level of consciousness.

Although heat itself is yang, a patient affected by summer heat may demonstrate yin symptoms if he has been drinking large amounts of cold fluids during his exposure to the harmful Chi of summer heat. In such a case the symptoms would include a feeling of coldness, headache, abdominal pain, and vomiting—the sort of symptoms that in the West are usually put down to a summer "tummy bug."

Heat itself is usually divided into three degrees of severity: fire (the most severe), heat, and mild heat. Fire can damage the mind, causing loss of consciousness or coma. Heat can combine with some of the other external factors in an invasion of the body, and diseases may be diagnosed as being due to damp heat, dry heat, or heat and wind. In addition, any of the other five external factors may, if very severe, develop into heat and combine heat symptoms with those of their own.

Many diseases that would be diagnosed by Chinese practitioners as due to heat are understood by Western doctors as acute infections, with their common symptoms of fever, thirst, and profuse sweating. Local infections, such as boils or abscesses, are also considered to be heat induced, since they are red, hot, and painful. When it invades the meridians, heat is said to drive out the blood that circulates there with the Chi and so may cause hemorrhage. For example, a patient with a severe intestinal infection who was passing bloody stools would be diagnosed as having had his Large Intestine meridian invaded by heat.

Heat can combine with wind to produce severe muscular spasms and convulsions associated with a high fever. If the patient remains untreated, he may finally become delirious and lapse into a coma. Dryness combined with heat will severely affect the lungs and will cause coughing together with spitting of blood. I said earlier that tuberculosis could be ascribed to an invasion by dryness that produces a dry cough and a wasting of the body. At a later stage of the disease, the patient may start to cough up blood; this would be diagnosed as due to heat that developed from the dryness when the latter became increasingly severe. Summer heat may increase in severity and turn into fire, which will exacerbate the symptoms that it has already caused.

THE SEVEN EMOTIONAL FACTORS

As we have seen, diseases of the types caused by the harmful external factors can also arise from within the body. Another way in which disease arises from within is as a result of the seven emotional factors. These can wear away the body's protective Chi, leaving the patient defenseless. The factors—joy, anger, melancholy, obsessional thinking, grief, fear, and fright—have to be very intense or very persistent in order to produce disease. When they are this severe, they often damage the internal organs: Anger is said to injure the liver, fright and joy the heart, grief and melancholy the lungs, obsessional thinking the spleen, and fear the kidneys. In some books obsessional thinking is referred to as meditation. However, true meditation and obsessional thinking are poles apart. It should not be thought that meditation, as practiced in many religions, particularly those of Eastern origin, can harm the spleen—or any other organ!

The emotion of anger has a number of yang attributes such as suddenness, heat, energy of movement, and the externalization of the angry person's emotions; it is therefore predominantly yang in character. Its arousal will produce yang symptoms similar to those produced by heat. If the liver—predominantly a yin organ—suffers physical damage as a result of attack by excessive yang, the patient may develop pain and swelling below his right-side ribs. The liver, in traditional Chinese thought, is responsible for keeping the meridians open and so allowing an unhindered flow of Chi around the body. It is also thought to be responsible for storing blood. Disruption of its function can thus produce hemorrhage (associated, as we have seen, with heat-induced disease) and menstrual problems. Depression and irritability are also said to result from injury to the liver.

The heart may be damaged by fright—in other words a sudden, severe shock—or by excessive joy. Either can cause the patient to develop palpitations, anxiety, insomnia, and mental disorders, since the heart is the seat of the mind. A Western physician, too, would agree that a sudden shock could cause all these symptoms, although he is unlikely to accept the idea that anxiety, insomnia, and mental problems have anything to do with the heart. Still, he would agree that a heart attack could be precipitated in a susceptible person by an extreme shock—or occasionally even by excessive joy and excitement. Patients who have severe angina (intermittent chest pain caused by an inadequate supply of blood to the muscles of the heart) are just as likely to develop pain as a result of watching an exciting football game or meeting up with a long-lost friend as they are from becoming angry or upset.

Fright is a sudden, severe, short-term emotion, while fear is more insidious and long term and must be persistent in order to produce disease. Fear is said to injure the kidney, which is the seat of willpower. Conversely, if the kidney is deficient in functional Chi—which is essential for its normal working—the patient is likely to be susceptible to fear.

Injury to the spleen, which is seen as a part of the digestive system, may occur as a result of obsessional thinking or constant worrying. This may cause anorexia (loss of appetite) and a feeling of abdominal distension, especially after meals. Western medicine recognizes the mental state of obsessional neurosis in which patients quite commonly number depression and anorexia among their symptoms. Indeed, anorexia nervosa may be thought of as a form of obsession.

Grief and melancholy (the latter includes anxiety) are said to affect the lung and therefore may interfere with breathing. In Western medicine it is known that anxiety may cause chronic overbreathing or hyperventilation, and that patients who suffer from panic attacks can be helped to control them by learning to control their breathing. Anxiety can also be a significant contributory factor to asthmatic attacks in susceptible patients. When hypnotherapy is used to treat asthmatic patients, one of the ways in which it works is to relieve the anxiety that the patient feels at the onset of an attack and so stop the vicious circle in which both anxiety and breathing problems steadily get worse as they feed on each other.

THE FOUR MISCELLANEOUS FACTORS

As well as the external and the emotional factors, disease may be due to four miscellaneous factors. Of these, the first three—irregular eating, excessive stress or lack of physical exercise, and trauma—are also accepted causes of disease in Western medicine, although the symptoms they are said to produce may not be the same. The fourth of the miscellaneous factors is stagnant blood and phlegm.

Irregular eating is a term that includes every form of bad eating habit, such as overeating, undereating, and excessive indulgence in alcohol, fat, or spices. It also includes eating food that is going bad or has been poisoned, and food that has little nutritional value (such as the junk foods so popular in the West).

Overeating is said to interfere with the function of the stomach and the spleen, both of which are intimately concerned in the digestive process. This can cause nausea, vomiting, belching, heartburn, distension, abdominal pain, and diarrhea. Since food is an important source of Chi, undereating can produce a deficiency in the body's Chi, causing weakness, dizziness, and emaciation. Unwholesome or poor-quality food will interfere with the function of the stomach and spleen, producing symptoms similar to those caused by overeating. Like Western medicine, Chinese medicine recognizes unwholesome food to be a cause of intestinal parasitic diseases. Excessive indulgence in alcohol, fat, and spices will stimulate the production of damp heat within the body, which may injure the vital organs. Western doctors would agree that alcohol in excess may damage the liver, while a very fatty diet can damage the heart.

Long-term stress or overexertion is said to use up the body's protective Chi and so leave it open to attack by the harmful external factors. It may cause weight loss, exhaustion, dizziness, and palpitations—symptoms also associated with excessive stress in the West. Lack of physical exercise can also lower the body's resistance to invasion, however, since it inhibits the flow of Chi and blood around the body and can therefore produce symptoms of weakness, exhaustion, shortness of breath, and—as recognized in the West—obesity.

Stagnant blood is said to have left the blood vessels and is therefore no longer circulating around the body. Instead it is retained in the tissues or in body cavities, and it causes symptoms wherever it accumulates. Commonly it causes pain that may be stabbing or boring in character, or sometimes colicky (waxing and waning in severity), but the area affected remains constant because the blood, being stagnant, does not move. Hemorrhage (either externally or into the skin) and bruising may also be symptoms of stagnant blood. When hemorrhage occurs, it is usually dark in color and may contain dark clots, unlike hemorrhage caused by heat, which tends to be a brighter red. Masses, tumors, and swelling of the internal organs may also be caused by stagnant blood.

Phlegm—the sticky fluid coughed up from the lungs of people with chest infections—is lumped together with stagnant blood in the list of miscellaneous factors, not because the two conditions necessarily occur together but because both have stagnant qualities. According to classical Chinese theory, phlegm can affect any part of the body, not just the lung, and is said to form when the body's use of water is abnormal. Excessive water accumulates within the body and is turned into phlegm, which may invade the organs or the meridians; here, because of its stickiness, it may completely block the flow of Chi. Such a blockage can be the cause of paralysis coupled with numbness, or with difficulty in speaking and distortion of the face, such as may occur in a patient who has had a stroke. Phlegm may, of course, affect the lung causing asthma or a severe cough in which the patient brings up large amounts of sputum. It may affect the stomach, producing abdominal distension and allowing fluid to collect in the abdominal cavity. If it attacks the heart—the seat of the mind—its capacity for causing blockages may result in the patient going into a coma. The rattle sometimes heard in the throat of a deeply comatose patient is said to be due to the phlegm lying there. Various soft, movable, superficial lumps—which in Western medicine might be diagnosed as cysts or lipomas (fat nodules), for example—are said to be due to accumulations of phlegm under the skin.

THE BASIS OF DIAGNOSIS

A diagnosis in acupuncture must be very exact: The more precise it is, the more likely the treatment is to be successful. Good treatment is based on good diagnosis. A trained acupuncturist will use the four basic techniques put together by Pien Chueh in the fourth century B.C.—observation, listening and smelling, questioning, and pulse diagnosis (this will be covered more fully in the next chapter). Based on this examination he will be able to decide which causative factor is responsible for the illness and how it has affected the body in terms of the meridians and the organs. On the basis of his findings he can separate diseases into certain well-defined groups, each associated with one of the Eight Principles. The characteristics associated with individual meridians may indicate which of these are involved in the disease state, and the symptoms may also indicate that certain of the internal, or zang-fu, organs have been affected. The way in which the disease has spread through the body from one meridian to another is the province of the Law of the Five Elements, which I covered in the previous chapter.

THE EIGHT PRINCIPLES

The Eight Principles are made up of four pairs of opposites: exterior and interior, cold and hot, xu (deficiency) and shi (excess), and yin and yang.

The conditions that they cause are sometimes referred to as *syndromes* (a Western medical term meaning "a collection of symptoms that occur together"). The four groups of principles are not mutually exclusive; so you may have, for example, a cold xu syndrome or a hot yang syndrome.

External and *internal* refer to the parts of the body that are affected and, to a certain extent, indicate the severity of the disease, since those that are internal are more serious than those that are external. For example, a skin disease or a mild infection such as a head cold is external, while a disease that attacks the core of the patient's well-being, such as pneumonia, is internal.

Cold and *hot* refer to the nature of the disease. Cold and hot syndromes exhibit symptoms that are associated with an invasion of the body by cold or by heat. In a *xu* (deficiency) syndrome, the protective Chi of the body is deficient and has therefore been powerless to prevent an invasion by harmful Chi. In a *shi* (excess) syndrome, however, the protective Chi is normal but has been overwhelmed by more powerful harmful Chi.

External, hot, and shi syndromes are by their nature predominantly *yang* in character, while internal, cold, and xu syndromes are predominantly *yin*. However, it is possible to have cold external syndromes, hot internal syndromes, external xu syndromes, internal shi syndromes, cold shi syndromes, and hot xu syndromes. Thus while it is possible to divide all diseases into yin types and yang types, it is important to remember that yin and yang are not concrete things but descriptions of the balance between two sides of a whole.

Since external syndromes are predominantly yang, they often develop suddenly and are short lived. Internal syndromes, on the other hand, are more likely to be long term. An external syndrome that is untreated or against which the body cannot defend itself may become more severe and move inward to become an internal syndrome. For example, an elderly or frail person who catches a head cold that then moves into the chest and turns into pneumonia may be seen as suffering from an external syndrome that has become internal. An internal syndrome may also be due to an intrinsic disorder of the internal zang-fu organs.

Cold syndromes and hot syndromes, as we have seen, are associated with the sort of symptoms that are caused by invasion by external cold and heat. Cold syndromes, being predominantly yin, are more likely to be long term than hot syndromes, which frequently take the form of acute infections. Xu syndromes, too, being "empty" and therefore yin, are inclined to be long term compared with the more acute shi syndromes.

The concept that an internal syndrome is always more serious than an external one is also found in homeopathy. Hering's Law of Cure—a homeopathic creed—states that illness is cured from the top down and from the inside out. So a homeopath would say that a patient who has eczema and then develops mild asthma is getting worse, even if his eczema has cleared up. However, a patient with asthma who stops having breathing problems is said to be getting better even if he has developed a very severe eczema. The eczema would be seen as an externalization of his problem, which is an essential step in its cure. Exactly the same is true with acupuncture treatment. A patient who has been suffering from an internal disease may have to trade in his symptoms for those of an external disease before he is finally cured.

In Chinese terms a common head cold, with its symptoms of runny nose, shivering, and mild fever, could be classified as a cold external syndrome. However, a diagnosis of a cold internal syndrome would be made on a patient who showed signs of coldness, pale skin, diarrhea, high fever, and general prostration—symptoms that even in Western terms would be associated with a far more serious condition, probably produced by a rampant infection.

A hot external syndrome is associated with a slight fever and sweating—the sort of symptoms you might expect to see in a mild case of flu. In a hot internal syndrome, however, you would find that the patient has a high fever, severe thirst, restlessness, a flushed face, constipation, and scanty urine. This is the sort of picture you might see in a disease such as scarlet fever, a far more serious condition than flu.

Certain types of flu that include headache and generalized aching in addition to the mild fever might be diagnosed as external shi syndromes.

Internal shi syndromes, however, present the sort of picture associated with a more serious chest infection: congestion in the chest associated with difficulty in breathing, malaise, and constipation.

Shi syndromes, with their predominantly yang characteristics, are (like external syndromes) usually acute and of sudden onset. They are often associated with fever, flushing of the face, and restlessness. The patient may complain of chestiness, abdominal pain, or difficulty in passing water, all reflecting the excess or "full" nature of the condition. A kidney infection might be classified as a shi syndrome based on symptoms of fever, abdominal pain of sudden onset, and pain on passing water.

Xu syndromes, which are predominantly yin, are inclined to be long standing. They are associated with the sort of symptoms you might expect in a disease where the life force is deficient: listlessness, apathy, poor memory, insomnia, shallow breathing and shortness of breath, poor vision, and incontinence. Sadly, these are all symptoms common in the elderly, chronically ill patient.

Having ascertained the type of syndrome from which his patient is suffering, the acupuncturist then has to decide which parts of the body are primarily affected. This will be based on his knowledge of the meridians and of the zang-fu organs. Symptoms may relate to an individual meridian—particularly when they are localized—and may be associated with the course of that meridian through the body or with the organ to which it is related. (Symptoms specifically associated with each of the twelve major meridians were mentioned in the previous chapter.)

Certain types of diseases are attributed to disruption, by various factors, of the functioning of the vital organs. It may sound as though this localization of diagnosis to a meridian or to an organ is akin to the Western practice of diagnosing in terms of a diseased part, but this is not the case. An acupuncture diagnosis says not that a particular meridian or organ is physically diseased but that its flow of energy has been disrupted, affecting its function. And the disruption, because it is one of energy, will have an effect not just on the organ or meridian itself but on the whole body.

THE ZANG-FU ORGANS

The functions attributed to the organs by Western medicine, such as the heart's role in the circulation of the blood and the kidney's role in the production of urine, are not the only ones recognized by the Chinese. For them the organs also have other, more subtle, functions in the maintenance of health. The heart, for example, is said to be the seat of the mind or spirit, and disruption of its function will affect the level of consciousness. Each of the zang (solid) organs is linked by one channel to a fu (hollow) organ and, by another channel, to a sense organ. Disruption of the Chi of a zang organ can affect the fu organ that is related to it. Similarly, the disruption of a fu organ's Chi will have an effect on its associated zang organ.

THE HEART

The heart, which is a zang organ, is linked to the small intestine (a fu organ) and the tongue (a sense organ). A long illness may affect the heart by causing a general weakness of Chi. If the Chi of the heart is weak, this will affect the organ's mechanical function, and the heart may develop irregularities in its beat. As a result the patient may suffer from palpitations and shortness of breath, especially upon exertion—symptoms that the Western physician, too, will associate with heart disease. If the weakness of Chi is not treated, it may develop into a general deficiency of its active aspect, yang, resulting in yin-associated symptoms such as a general lack of energy, coldness, and pallor, together with a susceptibility to other illnesses.

Conversely, if the yin of the heart becomes deficient, the symptoms produced may be due to the relative excess of yang. In this case the patient may be restless and feverish and have a flushed face. The deficiency of yin interferes with the function of the heart and thus of the mind that is housed there; it may cause insomnia, nightmares, poor memory, or other mental symptoms.

A long illness may weaken the heart, in turn interfering with its normal function of pumping blood around the body. A Chinese diagnostician would then say that there was stagnant blood in the heart, which was causing the symptoms and signs demonstrated by the patient: pain in the chest, palpitations, blue lips, and blue nails. This corresponds to Western medical thinking to the extent that an orthodox practitioner would recognize these as symptoms of inadequate circulation resulting from poor heart function, although he would not accept the Chinese concept of stagnant blood.

Severe heat, or fire, can also affect the heart. This can arise internally as a result of persistent mental problems that depress the body's Chi and stimulate the production of fire. The symptoms may include fever (reflecting the causative agent), insomnia (due to the effect on the mind, which is housed in the heart), and problems affecting the mouth and tongue, such as ulceration, pain, and swelling. The latter are due to fire affecting those parts of the body with which the heart is directly linked.

THE LIVER

The functions of the liver are said to be those of storing blood, maintaining the flow of Chi around the body, and keeping the tendons in good working order. The fu organ to which the liver is linked is the gallbladder (as, indeed, it is anatomically); Chi runs from the end of the Gall Bladder meridian into the start of the Liver meridian. The sense organ to which the liver is linked is the eye, and it is therefore associated with vision and with the maintenance of normal eyesight.

The functional Chi of the liver may become depressed, leading to stagnation of Chi in the Liver meridian. The initial depression of Chi can arise as a result of mental problems. Stagnant Chi may go on to produce stagnation of the blood, which may cause menstrual problems. If the Chi in the Liver meridian becomes blocked, the patient develops pain below the ribs and in the abdomen, with swelling of the abdomen and sometimes of the breasts. Here again there is a link with Western medical diagnosis, since patients who are diagnosed with cirrhosis of the liver not uncommonly have ascites (swelling of the abdomen due to an accumulation of fluid) and gynecomastia (swelling of the breasts) as well.

Severe heat, or fire, affecting the liver can be due to an overindulgence in alcohol or to excessive smoking; it may also be secondary to depression of the liver's Chi. The fire prevents Chi from flowing normally and, as a result, the patient may suffer from dizziness, headache, and irritability and may develop an inflammation of the eyes. If the blood stored by the liver becomes affected by the fire, hemorrhage may result, manifesting as nosebleeds or as vomiting of blood.

Heat can be associated with wind in an attack on the liver; in this case, the symptoms produced are attributable to both these external factors. The patient develops a high fever and may have convulsions possibly associated with neck rigidity and, later, coma. These are symptoms recognized in Western medicine as being due to an infection affecting the central nervous system—meningitis or encephalitis.

Cold may affect the liver and cause stagnation of Chi, particularly in the Liver meridian itself. This causes abdominal pain and, if the patient is male, can produce swelling and pain in the testicles, since the meridian runs through this area.

The liver is seen as a storehouse for blood, so chronic disease or hemorrhage, which are said to use up those stores, will produce a deficiency. As a result the body is no longer adequately nourished. Other functions of the liver will also be affected. There may be spasms in the tendons and muscles, which depend on the liver for their normal function, and the patient may have disturbances of vision, such as blurring and dizziness, and his eyes may feel dry and gritty. If the patient is female, her menstrual cycle can be affected, with her periods becoming scanty and irregular.

THE SPLEEN

The spleen is credited by the Chinese with control of digestion. It is said to be responsible for the proper absorption of nutrients from the ingested food and for their distribution around the body, so it is intimately linked with the stomach and its functions. As we saw in chapter 2, the beginning of the Spleen meridian follows on from the end of the Stomach meridian and receives Chi directly from it. The sense organ to which the spleen is linked is the mouth, although the tongue is associated with the heart. The spleen is also said to control the blood, ensuring that it remains within the blood vessels, and to be responsible for the maintenance of healthy muscles.

Because the spleen is involved in the extraction of Chi from food, it will naturally be affected by your eating habits. Irregular eating will cause the spleen's functional Chi to be weakened. Such a weakness may also be due to chronic stress or to long-term illness, giving rise to a poor appetite and inadequate food intake. If its own functional Chi is weak, the spleen will be unable to extract Chi adequately from what little food is being eaten, so that a vicious circle is set up. The patient develops lassitude, a sallow complexion, and diarrhea due to the overall deficiency of body nutrition. The muscles are no longer maintained in good condition, so the body loses its firmness; prolapse of the uterus or rectum (back passage) may occur. Blood is not properly contained within the blood vessels, which may result in spontaneous bruising or hemorrhage.

Because of its intimate association with the stomach and digestion, the spleen is susceptible to injury from any form of unbalanced diet. If excessive amounts of raw or cold food are eaten, this may open the spleen to attack from cold and damp. Again, this will be associated with poor appetite, and the patient may develop abdominal pain and diarrhea. Because cold is inclined to cause stagnation, the flow of Chi may become blocked and cause swelling in the upper abdomen, associated with lassitude and a heavy feeling in the head.

THE LUNGS

The lungs are, naturally, in charge of respiration. In addition to bringing oxygen into the body and expelling carbon dioxide, respiration takes in clean Chi and gets rid of waste Chi. The lungs are also said to control the use of water in the body and to maintain the health of the skin and the hair. The Lung meridian is coupled in the twenty-four-hour cycle with one of the other water-controlling meridians, the Urinary Bladder, so that when one is at its highest point in terms of the flow of Chi, the other is at its lowest. The lungs also link with the large intestine (since Chi flows from the Lung meridian into the Large Intestine meridian). The sense organ with which it is connected is of course the nose.

Chronic lung disease from whatever cause may result in a deficiency of the lung's yin. This affects the lung's control of the body's water and results in a dry mouth, fever, night sweats, and a dry cough, sometimes with some blood being coughed up. In Western terms these are all symptoms that may be associated with a diagnosis of tuberculosis. I mentioned earlier that the symptoms of tuberculosis could be produced by an invasion of the lungs by heat and dryness—both predominantly yang factors whose long-term presence can result in a chronic deficiency of yin.

The lungs can also be affected by wind, which may be accompanied by cold. The wind produces a cough and a blocked nose, while the additional cold may aggravate the condition, causing a sensation of coldness, a nasal discharge, and the coughing up of sputum. These are symptoms that are often associated with the common cold. If the invading wind is accompanied by heat, the symptoms are those of a rather more severe form of the infection, with fever, sore throat, and purulent nasal discharge and sputum.

If the body's use of water—controlled by the lungs—becomes disrupted, fluid can accumulate within the lung as damp or phlegm. This in turn blocks the flow of Chi, and the patient becomes short of breath and brings up a lot of white sputum. Phlegm may also develop as a result of the invasion of the lung by wind and heat. This too will block the flow of Chi so that the patient develops a cough with shortness of breath. In this case, because the phlegm is hot, blood stagnates; as a result the sputum that is brought up is not only copious but also purulent.

THE KIDNEYS

As well as having a role in maintaining the body's water balance, the kidneys are said to be in charge of reproduction, growth, and development. Although these last three are not functions associated with the kidneys in Western medicine, it is interesting to note that they may be associated with the adrenal glands—which are situated immediately above the kidneys on the back wall of the abdominal cavity. The adrenals produce steroid hormones, and disruption of their function may produce abnormalities of growth and development as well as interfering with normal reproduction. The adrenals also secrete the hormones that regulate the kidneys' function of excreting water.

In Chinese medicine the kidneys work together with the lungs in their capacity of controlling the body's use of water. The kidneys are also said to regulate the distribution around the body of clean Chi, extracted from the inhaled air by the lungs. They are responsible for the formation of the bone marrow, the blood, and the brain, which is considered a specialized form of marrow. They are linked to the bladder (as it is anatomically), since the end of the Urinary Bladder meridian opens into the start of the Kidney meridian. The sense organ with which they are associated is the ear, and deafness in the elderly is said to be due to a deficiency of functional Chi in the kidneys.

Long-term illness can weaken the kidneys' Chi. Such weakness may also occur congenitally, or it may be due to senility. Whatever the cause, symptoms associated with urination are likely to occur, including an increase in frequency, dribbling, or incontinence. The reproductive system may be affected, resulting in infertility. Because the kidneys are associated with and works together with the lungs, weakness of its functional Chi may also cause shortness of breath or asthma.

A deficiency of yin or yang, either of which may occur as the result of a long illness, may have an effect on the kidneys. It is said that such a deficiency can also be due to an overindulgence in sexual activity. If yin is deficient, the patient may experience dizziness, blurring of vision, poor memory, and tinnitus (ringing in the ears) due to the kidneys' inability to maintain the normal functions of the brain and of the ears. Since a deficiency of yin necessarily results in a relative excess of yang, yang-type symptoms such as feverishness and night sweats will occur.

Yang's association with activity means that a deficiency of yang in the kidneys will lead to a reduction in the activity of the kidneys. This can cause fluid retention and failure to pass adequate amounts of urine. The reduction in activity may also affect bladder function, resulting in problems such as dribbling and retention of urine. In addition, the relative excess of yin will cause pallor and symptoms of coldness; a male patient may become impotent.

THE PERICARDIUM

The pericardium may be invaded by heat. This will produce symptoms of high fever, delirium, and coma as a result of the effect on the mind, which is housed in the heart.

THE GALLBLADDER

Jaundice is said to be caused by an invasion of the gallbladder by damp heat. This may be due to a primary malfunction in the liver or to long-term overindulgence in alcohol or rich food. Because damp causes stagnation, the flow of Chi is impaired; the resulting blockage prevents bile from being excreted freely. Thus the patient develops jaundice and may vomit bile. It is the blockage of Chi in the gallbladder and the liver that produces the pain many jaundiced patients experience in the upper right part of their abdomens.

THE STOMACH

Overeating may disrupt the functional Chi of the stomach, causing food to be retained within it. This will result in distension and pain in the upper abdomen, together with belching, nausea, and vomiting.

Ingesting large amounts of raw or cold food may cause the stomach to be attacked by cold. This can also occur if the patient gets soaked by cold rain. The invading cold causes stagnation of the functional Chi of the stomach, resulting in the retention of fluid and causing pain and swelling in the upper abdomen and, sometimes, vomiting. Similar symptoms may also be due to depression of the stomach's yang, which may occur after a long illness. The deficiency of active yang together with a relative excess of yin are the factors that cause the stagnation in this case. Eating large quantities of rich food can cause heat to accumulate in the stomach, resulting in a burning pain in the upper abdomen, thirst, vomiting, and foul breath.

THE LARGE INTESTINE

Although it lies farther along the digestive tract than the stomach, the large intestine may also have its function disrupted by dietary abnormalities. Eating excessive amounts of raw, cold, or unwholesome food may cause the large intestine to be affected by damp heat. The damp causes stagnation and thus hinders the normal flow of Chi. As a result the patient develops diarrhea and abdominal pain. The heat may cause hemorrhage, which shows itself as blood in the stools. These are symptoms that Western doctors, too, would associate with food poisoning.

Disruption of the flow of Chi in the large intestine may also be due to stagnation of the blood flow, causing constipation, abdominal pain, and distension. A more serious version of this may be caused by an invasion of the large intestine by heat due to overeating or a particular susceptibility of the patient to weather changes. This can cause inflammation of the intestine and the formation of abscesses in addition to the symptoms already mentioned.

THE BLADDER

Damp heat may invade the bladder and cause the sort of symptoms that are associated in Western medicine with infections of the urinary tract, including frequent passing of water with associated burning and pain. The heat can also cause hemorrhage and consequent passage of blood in the urine. If the condition is not treated, the damp may give rise to stagnation, which in turn may result in the formation of stones.

5

Methods of Diagnosis

The experienced acupuncturist's familiar knowledge of the functions of the meridians and of the zang-fu organs will enable him to assess which of these has had its flow of Chi disrupted and in what manner. However, he will also use pulse and tongue diagnosis to decide how this disruption has been brought about, and in addition may look at the patient's face, skin, and general appearance, and ask him about his eating and sleeping habits, urine, and bowels. From all of this the acupuncturist will be able to determine whether the patient is suffering from a xu (deficiency) syndrome or a shi (excess) syndrome, whether yin or yang is predominant, and which of the external, emotional, or miscellaneous factors may be responsible for the illness.

THE PULSE

The radial artery, which runs across the wrist, is used by both Chinese and Western physicians when they take a pulse, but their methods are quite different. Chinese pulse diagnosis is a very exact science, far removed from the simple counting of beats practiced in the West, and it may take a student many years of practice before he is proficient at it. Students who have only attended short courses in acupuncture have learned no more than the very basics of pulse diagnosis and will usually rely mainly on the condition of the tongue to back up their diagnosis. Although tongue diagnosis will give the same indications as pulse diagnosis, it is not nearly as accurate. The difference between a practitioner using only tongue diagnosis and one who combines this with pulse diagnosis may be compared with the difference between two Western doctors, one armed with a stethoscope and blood pressure equipment and the other with an electrocardiogram (EKG) machine as well. The first doctor can quite easily diagnose a patient who has had a heart attack from the symptoms that are presented and from the signs that he can observe using his equipment. However, the doctor with the EKG machine will be able to tell which part of the heart has been affected and how severe the heart attack has been. He will also be able to monitor, on an hour-to-hour basis, any improvement or deterioration in his patient's condition.

When a Western physician takes a pulse, he puts his fingers lightly on one of the patient's wrists and feels the radial artery somewhere along the stretch where it runs just under the skin. A Chinese physician, while using the same stretch of the same artery, will feel it at six well-defined places on each wrist, three superficial and three deep. Each of these pulses reflects the condition of one of the twelve major meridians and their associated organs, allowing their balance to be assessed, while the character of the pulse as a whole indicates the type of syndrome affecting the patient. Comparing each pulse against the others allows any sign of excess or deficiency in a particular meridian to be detected.

All the superficial pulses are associated with the fu (hollow) organs and their meridians, which are predominantly yang. On the right wrist are the pulses that are linked to the large intestine, stomach, and sanjiao, while on the left are those linked to the small intestine, gallbladder, and urinary bladder. The deep pulses are associated with the zang (solid) organs, which are predominantly yin: the lung, spleen, and pericardium on the right, and the heart, liver, and kidney on the left.

However, this is not the end of the story where yin and yang are concerned. Left-sidedness is associated with yin and right-sidedness with yang, so all the pulses on the left wrist reflect the total yin of the body and all those on the right wrist the yang. If all the pulses on the right are normal but those on the left are stronger, this indicates an excess of yin; the reverse indicates an excess of yang. Similarly, normal pulses on the right combined with weak pulses on the left suggest a deficiency of yin, while a deficiency of yang would present as normal pulses on the left and weak pulses on the right.

We have already seen that the aspects of yin and yang are not concrete but fluctuate according to how they are looked at; this applies just as much to pulse diagnosis as to anything else. An outer or exterior position is always predominantly yang compared with an inner position, which is predominantly yin. The outer pulses are those that are closest to the wrist (and therefore farthest from the heart), while the inner pulses are those slightly higher up the arm. If the outer pulses (relating to the large intestine and lung on the right, the small intestine and heart on the left) are stronger than the inner pulses (sanjiao and pericardium on the right, urinary bladder and kidney on the left), this indicates a relative excess of yang in the body. If, however, the inner pulses are stronger, a relative excess of yin is indicated. The balance of yin and yang can also be determined by comparing the superficial and the deep pulses, since deepness is yin while superficiality is yang.

Having determined the balance of yin and yang and the balance among the organs and meridians, the acupuncturist will then assess the quality of the pulse in order to elicit further information as to the type of syndrome affecting his patient. Numerous qualities of pulse have been described, although many of these categories appear to run into each other and their fine distinctions are perceived only by the expert. However, for our purposes, they may be divided into a few broadly based groups.

The first of these is the *rapid pulse,* which is defined as having more than five beats to a breath (note that in Chinese medicine the pulse is timed by the patient's breathing and not by the doctor's watch). A rapid pulse often occurs when there is an excess of yang and therefore increased activity in the body, or when the patient is suffering from a hot syndrome. This tallies with Western diagnosis, in which a rapid pulse (albeit timed by the clock) may be associated with a fever.

The rapid pulse may be either *forceful* or *weak,* a forceful quality indicating an excess of Chi or a shi syndrome, whereas a weak pulse would be indicative of a xu (deficiency) syndrome.

Cold syndromes are associated with a *slow pulse,* also measured according to the patient's breathing. Less than four beats to the breath is categorized as slow. As with a rapid pulse, forcefulness suggests a shi syndrome, while a weak pulse implies a xu syndrome.

There is, as you would expect, a strong correlation between the Chinese concept of a normal pulse rate—between four and five beats to the breath—and that held by physicians in the West. In the West, where the pulse is measured as number of beats per minute, the norm is around seventy-two, while the normal number of breaths per minute is around sixteen. Divide the normal pulse rate by the normal breath rate, and you come up with four and a half, the midway point of the Chinese normal range.

If an excess or a deficiency of Chi occurs without the involvement of cold or heat, as in a shi or xu syndrome, this can also be diagnosed from the pulse. A xu pulse feels weak when pressed lightly and disappears completely on heavy pressure, whereas a shi pulse feels forceful whether you press lightly or firmly. A thready pulse may also indicate a xu syndrome, while a large bounding pulse may occur in a shi syndrome.

External and internal syndromes also have their own diagnostic types of pulse. External syndromes may be indicated, in the early stages, by a *superficial* or *floating pulse.* This is a pulse that is readily felt when the pressure exerted is light but becomes weak if pressed hard. It gives a sensation of floating on the surface of the skin. A fine distinction of this type of pulse is one that conveys the floating feeling and yet is either weak or forceful. If it is weak, it suggests that the patient is suffering from a long-term illness and a deficiency of yang. A forceful floating pulse, however, would be associated with an external syndrome in which there was an excess of yang.

A *deep pulse* is the diagnostic opposite of a floating pulse. It is necessary to exert increased pressure in order to feel this pulse, which is associated with internal syndromes. Again, it may be forceful or weak, force being associated with an excess and weakness with a deficiency.

Sometimes a pulse is described as being *slippery* or *gliding*, feeling almost as though it is wriggling under the fingers and often compared to ball bearings rolling on a plate. This type of pulse is an indication that phlegm is causing problems. When the pulse is forceful it suggests that the seat of the patient's problem is in the digestive tract. When it is weak it indicates that phlegm has accumulated due to a general weakness of the body. A full gliding pulse may also occur in healthy people, however, particularly during pregnancy.

A completely different quality of pulse, with none of the easy movement of the slippery pulse, is known as a *rough pulse*. It may occur in conditions of deficiency of Chi or blood, particularly if the kidney is affected, in which case it will be weak; or it may also indicate stagnation due to an invasion by cold damp, in which case it will be forceful.

An *irregular pulse* in Western medicine indicates an irregular heartbeat due to an electrical misfiring in the mechanism that regulates the contraction of the heart muscle. To a Chinese physician, it is an indication of stagnation of blood with interference to the flow of Chi and a deficiency of yang.

The *bowstring* or *wiry pulse* is hard and forceful, giving the impression of a tightly pulled string. While it may be found in a healthy person, it can also occur in a patient who is in pain or in one who has a deficiency of yin with a relative excess of yang in the liver.

Within these definitions, there are further divisions. For example, as well as the slow and rapid categories, varieties of rate and rhythm may be described as *knotted, intermittent, scattered, moving, hasty, slowing,* or *fast.*

THE TONGUE

Tongue diagnosis has fewer nuances than pulse diagnosis and takes less time to learn, but it is still of great value to the experienced practitioner of Chinese medicine. In Western medicine a healthy tongue is said to be pink and moist with little or no coating. This is also accepted as normal in Chinese medicine, but assessment of the tongue goes much farther than this. As with the pulse, the findings are expressed in terms of the cause of the patient's disease and the energy imbalances that have resulted.

A normal tongue is pink. Anything else is said to be abnormal. Abnormal colors are classified as pale, red, purplish red, or purple. A pale tongue, as you might guess, is indicative of a deficiency syndrome (particularly a deficiency of yang) or of a disease caused by cold. A deficiency of blood will also cause a pale tongue, which tallies with the Western acceptance of a pale tongue as one of the signs of anemia. If the tongue appears glossy and pale, it suggests that the problem is a long-standing one.

If the patient has a wet pale tongue, this indicates that the yang of the spleen is deficient. According to the Law of the Five Elements, the spleen is the master of the kidney. If the spleen is deficient (the paleness indicating deficiency), then it will be unable to control the kidney. This will affect the body's fluids, causing the tongue to become abnormally wet.

A red tongue is suggestive of a disease caused by heat or of a deficiency of yin, causing a relative excess of yang. A purplish red tongue occurs in acute diseases caused by heat, such as acute fevers. In such cases the tongue may also be dry, indicating that the body's fluids have been affected by the heat. A purplish red tongue can also occur in patients who, due to a prolonged and severe illness, are deficient in yin. In such a case it is likely to have a glossy appearance, signifying that there has been damage to both the yin and the body's fluids.

A purple tongue is recognized by Western doctors as associated with heart disease, particularly with heart failure and inadequate pumping of the blood around the body. In Chinese medicine it may indicate a stagnation of Chi and of blood. It may also occur if there is an excess of internal cold due to a deficiency of yang.

The coating of the tongue is said to be formed from food residues together with yang Chi derived from the spleen, and so it will reflect any abnormalities of the digestive system. Its color and condition are also indicative of various states occurring within the body. The coating may be described as white, yellow, grayish black, or peeled; in addition, it may be thin, thick, sticky, moist, or dry. A thick coating usually indicates a more serious problem than a thin coating of the same color. Patchy coating occurs when the spleen and stomach are not working together properly in the production of Chi. Moistness is suggestive of an invasion by damp, or of an imbalance in the body's fluids due to a deficiency in the yang of the kidney or spleen (its master according to the Law of the Five Elements). A dry coating is usually due to a deficiency of bodily fluids following an invasion by heat, and a sticky coating suggests that phlegm is the cause of the patient's condition.

A thin white coating may occur in a healthy person but, when seen in a patient suffering from a disease, it indicates an invasion of the lung by wind and cold. A thin yellow coating, on the other hand, is never normal and may mean that the lung has been invaded by wind and heat.

If the coating of the tongue is white and thick, it suggests that food is being retained. A more serious and long-term form of this is suggested by a thick yellow coating.

A sticky white coating indicates invasion by cold and damp or the retention within the body of phlegm and damp. It might be seen, for example, in a patient with bronchitis. A sticky yellow coating indicates retention of damp heat or a blockage in the lung caused by phlegm and heat, and might be seen in a patient suffering from a lung abscess.

A dry white coating to the tongue indicates invasion by a *pestilential factor*—a term used to include all forms of epidemic contagious diseases. A dry yellow coating reflects both heat and an imbalance of bodily fluids, suggesting an accumulation of heat in the stomach and intestines that has damaged yin and fluids.

A yellow coating may, of course, also be seen on the tongues of smokers, so an acupuncturist will always want to know whether or not his patient smokes. His pleasure on finding that a patient is a nonsmoker will be twofold: First, it will make his diagnosis easier, because the color of the tongue and its coating will not be masked; second, his treatment will not be counteracted by the patient continuing to assault his body with toxins!

The tongue may sometimes have a bald or peeled appearance. This is often associated, in Western terms, with a severe vitamin deficiency. To the Chinese physician, it may indicate a prolonged and severe illness in which the patient's protective Chi has been severely damaged and a considerable deficiency of yin has occurred—events that might be associated with malnutrition.

A moist grayish black coating on the tongue usually suggests that cold and damp have been retained within the body or that inner cold has welled up due to a deficiency of yang and a relative excess of yin. A grayish black coating that is dry and seen on a red tongue indicates a drying out of bodily fluids by excessive heat, which in turn may be due to a deficiency of yin with a relative excess of yang. This sort of tongue may occur in patients who, in Western terms, are dehydrated.

The tongue can, of course, be colored by things other than disease and smoking. Candy, soft drinks, and some fruits and vegetables can all stain the tongue, so it is important to ensure that you haven't dyed it in some new shade when you go to see your acupuncturist!

In addition to its color, the condition of the tongue can reveal important things to the practitioner about his patient's condition. A patient with a large and flabby tongue that is pale and perhaps shows the impression of his teeth around the edge is likely to be suffering from a general deficiency of Chi and yang and to have an accumulation within the body of phlegm and damp. If the tongue is flabby but red, this suggests an excess of heat that is affecting the stomach or the heart. A flabby purplish tongue occurs when there is stagnation of blood. A tongue that is a normal shade of pink may also be flabby; in this case it would suggest an accumulation of damp heat in the spleen or stomach, or a deficiency of yang.

A tongue that has fissures in it and looks cracked may be normal in some people, so if your tongue looks like this you may be asked whether it has always looked so. If, however, the cracks have only appeared with the onset of the illness, they may indicate a drying up of the body's fluids due to excessive heat, and a deficiency of yin in the kidney, with a relative excess of yang.

The tongue may display on its surface little bumps, which are usually red. These, too, suggest excessive heat with a drying up of bodily fluids, and may also indicate stagnation of the blood. This appearance is called a thorny tongue and it may be seen in a patient who has recently suffered from an infectious illness. White bumps on the tongue or flat purple blotches may occur in severe cases of invasion by heat, and the latter may also indicate stagnation of blood and of Chi.

A stiff and tremulous tongue is usually associated in Western medicine with some form of neurological disorder. In Chinese medicine it is an indication of a disturbance of the mind caused by phlegm and heat. The tongue is, of course, the sense organ that is linked to the heart, which is the seat of the mind. A stiff, tremulous tongue may also be seen in a patient suffering from a deficiency in the liver's yin due to an invasion by heat, or it may be associated with an obstruction of the collateral channels by wind and phlegm. When it is seen during a prolonged illness, it suggests an overall deficiency of Chi and of yin. A tongue that is deviated to one side of the mouth, such as may occur after a stroke, is also said to indicate obstruction of the collateral channels by wind and phlegm. Wind is often said to be the causative factor of a stroke.

Wind can cause blockages that interfere with both movement and sensation, so if a patient complains that his tongue feels numb, it may indicate that wind is a causative factor in his illness. This may have arisen either from a yin deficiency or—if the tongue is red—from an excess of Chi affecting the liver.

A thin tongue is said to indicate a deficiency syndrome. If the tongue is pale this suggests that the deficiency is one of Chi and of blood, whereas if it is red the deficiency is likely to be of yin, producing a relative excess of yang.

Tongue diagnosis and pulse diagnosis are the two most valuable diagnostic tools available to the acupuncturist, which is why I have gone into the details of both techniques before mentioning any others. When a you visit an acupuncturist, however, it is likely that your general appearance will be observed and that you'll be asked questions about yourself before any reference is made to your pulse or tongue.

HABITS AND OTHER SYMPTOMS AND SIGNS

In both Western and Chinese medicine the patient's habits may provide clues as to the problem affecting him and its cause. But the interpretation that an acupuncturist puts on the information that the patient provides will be quite different from that made by a Western physician. For example, a patient who has to stand a great deal in the course of his work may develop problems affecting the kidney and its meridian, while a patient who sits all day may have problems affecting the spleen. The spleen may also be affected by excessive concentration (a lesser degree of the obsessional thinking mentioned earlier), as may the stomach, with which it works in the digestion of food and extraction of Chi. You may see this sort of effect in the so-called workaholic who spends long hours at his desk, striving for perfection in his work, and ends up developing a peptic ulcer.

The patient's eating habits are important, too, as are his reactions to food. As we have seen, overeating or the consumption of junk foods may contribute to the development of disease, as may an excessive intake of spices, fat, or alcohol. If a patient feels better after he has eaten, this suggests that he is deficient in Chi—it is the Chi derived from the food he has just eaten that is giving him this temporary relief. Conversely, a patient whose symptoms increase in severity after he has eaten is likely to have an excess of Chi, with the Chi in the food making matters worse. If he feels bloated after eating, this suggests that the Chi he has extracted from the food is being prevented from circulating correctly and that there is stagnation. Constant thirst indicates a hot syndrome, while an absence of thirst suggests an invasion by cold or damp.

Certain tastes are associated with certain elements; when they appear abnormally, they may thus indicate problems relating to the organs or meridians linked to those elements. A sour taste is associated with wood, a bitter taste with fire, sweetness with earth, heat (as in curry) with metal, and saltiness with water. So a salty taste in the mouth may be a symptom of disturbance of the kidney (one of the water organs) by heat. Since the spleen is associated with earth, damp heat affecting the spleen may produce a sweet taste in the mouth. Heat affecting the fire-associated heart is likely to result in a bitter taste. A patient who has lost his sense of taste altogether is likely to have a deficiency of his spleen's functional Chi. Bad breath is a result of heat in the stomach.

A patient's illness may also be reflected in his sleeping patterns. Excessive sleepiness may be due to a deficiency of yang with a corresponding excess of the inactive principle, yin. Insomnia, on the other hand, may indicate a deficiency of yin in the liver and kidney or an overall deficiency of Chi. Early-morning waking suggests a deficiency of Chi, particularly in the Gall Bladder meridian, or it may be due to an excess of heat in the heart. The heart and gallbladder are also implicated if the patient is a very light sleeper, when a disturbance of the Chi of either may be involved.

Like a Western physician, an acupuncturist may question the patient about his urine and bowels. Here again, though, the conclusions that he draws from the answers will be different from the Western ones.

If the patient passes a lot of urine or has to get up at night to pass water, he is likely to have a deficiency in the kidney's yang. A total deficiency of Chi in the kidney and bladder, however, may reduce the amount of urine produced to below normal. Incontinence may also be caused by a deficiency of the kidney's functional Chi.

Blood in the urine may be an indication of damp heat in the bladder, heat being a common cause of hemorrhage. If the urine is a particularly dark yellow in color, this also suggests an invasion by heat, whereas pale urine indicates an invasion by cold or a deficiency of the kidney's yang, with a relative excess of yin.

The type of stools that the patient passes may indicate the state of his intestines. Since damp is associated with stagnation and foul-smelling discharges, the passage of watery, foul-smelling stools is a good indication that the intestines have been invaded by damp heat.

While the acupuncturist is interviewing the patient he will, like any Western physician, be observing him. If the patient appears apprehensive— or perhaps I should say more apprehensive than might be considered normal for a patient on his first visit to an acupuncturist—this may suggest a problem with the kidney, the urinary bladder, or their meridians. If the patient is tense, the liver and gallbladder may be implicated, while a patient whose attention wanders may have problems with the spleen or stomach. The kidney and urinary bladder may also be involved if the patient is overweight or has abnormally cold hands.

A great deal can be discovered by observing the patient's face. As with the tongue, the color can be very informative. A red face, of course, is suggestive of an invasion by heat. A sallow complexion indicates a deficiency, usually affecting the spleen (which is responsible for the extraction and circulation of Chi), and also suggests an invasion by damp. Damp heat in the spleen may produce a dark, orange-colored jaundice, while a lighter yellow jaundice may be due to damp cold.

A very pale complexion, too, may be associated with a total body deficiency of Chi or yang (such as might occur after a hemorrhage), or with a deficiency of Chi together with cold in the lungs. If the patient's face is pale but his cheeks and lips are red, a deficiency of yin may have resulted in the production of heat through the relative excess of yang.

Pale lips, like a pale complexion, signify a deficiency, particularly in the lung. Bright red lips, on the other hand, are indicative of heat, especially affecting the heart. Dry lips suggest that heat is affecting the spleen or that there is an imbalance of the body's fluids. The condition of the spleen is also implicated if the lips are swollen.

Red and painful eyes may indicate that the patient is suffering from an excess of yang and heat. If they itch, an invasion by wind and heat may have occurred. The organ with which the eyes are linked is the liver. If the kidney's yin is deficient and, as a result, it fails to nourish the liver (its "child" according to the Law of the Five Elements), the yin of the latter may also become deficient. This may be suspected if a patient complains that light hurts his eyes. A deficiency of Chi in the kidney, resulting in a deficiency in the liver, may produce double vision. Blurred vision, however, can be a result of an abnormality of the blood or of yin.

There are differing views as to the diagnostic value of lines and blemishes in various positions on the face. Some practitioners believe that the entire body is reflected in the face. Others, however, dispute the reliability of this type of diagnosis.

The condition of the skin and nails is more widely accepted as useful in diagnosis. Dry, flaky skin suggests that the circulation of Chi and blood is sluggish, leaving the skin inadequately nourished. If the skin becomes puffy, this may be due to a blockage in the flow of Chi, while a deficiency of Chi will result in the skin becoming thin and wrinkled. Nails that break easily or seem soft also suggest a deficiency of Chi or blood, particularly one affecting the liver (upon whose normal function the health of the nails depends).

Although the techniques of acupuncture and the ways in which diagnoses are made are so different from those used in Western medicine, a patient who visits an acupuncturist for the first time may well feel that his initial consultation was rather similar to one he might have had with his own family doctor. Many of the questions asked will be the same, and examinations of tongue, pulse, skin, and nails will have a familiar ring. And although Chinese and Western doctors will interpret the symptoms and signs presented to them very differently, in both cases it is on this interpretation and diagnosis that treatment will be based.

6

Methods of Treatment

In Western medicine both diagnosis and treatment are usually based upon a part of the body. For example, a diagnosis of a broken bone will be followed by treatment of that bone by putting it in plaster, and a diagnosis of an irregular heartbeat will be followed by treatment of the heart with drugs to regulate its rhythm. A patient diagnosed with gallstones is likely to have his gallbladder removed and, with it, the stones. However, removing a patient's gallstones does not treat their initial cause. While the stones do not re-form, since the gallbladder is no longer there, the imbalance that originally created them has not been cured by the operation.

In Chinese medicine the aim of treatment is not just to alleviate the illness itself but to do so by removing its cause. A patient whose illness is diagnosed as being due to an invasion by heat, no matter what his symptoms may be, will be given treatment aimed at dispelling heat from the body. Similarly, a patient with excessive yin will be treated so as to sedate yin and stimulate yang. It is of course sometimes possible to treat specific symptoms with acupuncture, since some acupuncture points have specific effects—to lower blood pressure, for instance, or stop vomiting. However, these points are not usually used as a complete treatment in themselves.

Acupuncture, like many other complementary therapies, is a way of restoring the body's energy flow to a normal state so that the body can get on with the work of healing itself. When there is a deficiency of Chi, yin, or yang, then, the system must be stimulated; when there is an excess it must be reduced. Heat, cold, wind, damp, dryness, or phlegm must be eliminated from the body, and stagnant blood must be set flowing again. Imbalances among the meridians must be remedied by drawing Chi into a deficient meridian from one that has excess. A mother meridian must be encouraged to nourish its child, and a master meridian must be adjusted so that it has appropriate control over its servant. If there is a blockage of Chi flowing along the course of a single meridian, this must be unblocked.

Each meridian's points have specific functions relating to the transfer of energy. The element points have already been mentioned in chapter 3. In addition, each meridian has a source point by which it is linked to its organ. Thus, the source point on the Lung meridian may be used to treat the lung itself, that on the Kidney meridian may be used to treat the kidney, and so on. Some points are specific for dispelling the various external factors: heat, wind, cold, damp, dryness, and summer heat. Others have particular effects on yin or yang, either stimulating or sedating. On each of the major meridians—except that of the heart—are one or more intersection or meridian connection points by which that meridian is linked to others. These points are useful for the treatment of conditions in which several meridians are affected.

Along the Urinary Bladder meridian, as it runs down the back, lies a series of points that have an effect on the other major meridians. These are known as the associated or shu points. Each meridian is related to one shu point lying between Urinary Bladder (UB) 13 and UB 28, parallel to the spine. On the front of the trunk are twelve similar alarm or mu points, which are also each connected to one of the major meridians. The mu points do not lie on a single meridian. Six of them (those relating to the Pericardium, Heart, Stomach, Sanjiao, Small Intestine, and Urinary Bladder meridians) are midline and are points on the Ren meridian. The others are bilateral. The Lung mu point, the Liver mu point, and the Gall Bladder mu point each lies on its own meridian, but the Kidney mu point lies on the Gall Bladder meridian, the Spleen mu point on the Liver meridian, and the Large Intestine mu point on the Stomach meridian. Both the mu and the shu points may be used diagnostically: If they become tender or painful, this indicates a disturbance involving their associated meridian.

The choice of points to be used in treatment is therefore very complicated. The acupuncturist must know the function of each of the points on each of the meridians, along with the nonmeridian extra points. He must know how the meridians interact with each other. He must know how to eliminate invasive conditions, such as cold and heat, from the body. He must know how to restore balance to the system and how to stimulate it to function normally once more. And, ideally, he must be able to do this while using a minimum of needles.

People are often worried at the thought of being stuck full of needles. But the skill of a trained acupuncturist lies in knowing how to treat a condition using the fewest possible acupuncture points. Often a patient may be treated with no more than four or five needles, and indeed, sometimes a single needle will be enough. Five correctly chosen points will produce results just as good as ten. In the next chapter a variety of illnesses is discussed, and a number of points listed that might be used in the treatment of each of them. In some cases there may be a large number of suitable points, but these would not all be used at the same time. However, where there is a wide range of equally appropriate points and where the treatment is carried out over a period of weeks or months, the practitioner might use all of them in rotation.

Of course, treatment need not necessarily involve the use of a needle. Although needling is probably the easiest, most effective, and therefore most popular way of stimulating the acupuncture points, it is not the only one. Other methods are widely used, both to complement acupuncture and in cases where needles are inappropriate (for example, in the treatment of young children).

Acupressure is the treatment of the acupuncture points by massage. Usually the pressure is pulsed, or applied and released a number of times. How long pressure is applied each time may depend on whether the point is tender. If it is, the therapist may press for only a second or two before resting. However, the patient will soon realize that, as treatment continues, the point becomes less tender; after a few uncomfortable minutes he will be able to withstand pressure applied to the point for longer and longer periods. Since a tender acupuncture point is an indication that the point needs treating, the diminution of the tenderness shows that the treatment is working. This can be very encouraging to both patient and therapist.

There are, however, three drawbacks to acupressure. First, only one point can be treated at a time (bilaterally if necessary), whereas more may be needed, particularly in patients with long-term problems. Second, the therapist obviously must remain with the patient throughout the treatment—unlike acupuncture where, once the needles are in, the patient can be left alone for a few minutes while they take effect. Third, the therapist needs to have very strong and resilient hands or he may find that he needs treatment himself—for painful thumbs!

In chapter 1 I mentioned that *moxibustion* can be useful in the treatment of conditions that tend to be more prevalent in a damp climate. Moxa is still used today to treat conditions caused by cold and damp and, as you might expect, is especially useful in areas such as Japan, Great Britain, and the Pacific Northwest. Certain points are particularly susceptible to treatment with moxa.

The usual method of using moxa is to attach a small wad of it to the end of an acupuncture needle that has been inserted into the relevant point. Once the moxa is lit, the warmth it produces travels down the needle and into the point. Since the shortest needle in common use is an inch long and has a handle that is also an inch long or more, the moxa is never less than about an inch and a half away from the skin. Thus the patient is unlikely to get scorched.

Cupping is another method of treating points that need warming in order to eliminate cold or damp. However, unlike moxibustion—which is applied to an individual point and can be used on any part of the body—cupping can only be used where there are large flat surfaces (such as the back or the thighs) wide enough to take the cups. The cups are made of glass or bamboo and are heated, usually by inserting a burning taper inside them, which creates a partial vacuum. The taper is removed and the cup is immediately placed onto the skin, where it adheres via the suction created by the vacuum.

The cups are left on the skin for a few minutes before they are gently pried off, often leaving raised pink marks. These marks usually disappear fairly rapidly. The suction produced by the cups is quite strong (this is what causes the pink marks, since blood is drawn into the surface vessels of the skin)—strong enough, it is said, to draw out the cold or damp causing the disease. Cupping is therefore very useful for conditions such as bronchitis where the acupuncturist has diagnosed an invasion by cold or damp and where the area affected—in this case the skin overlying the lung—can be covered using four to six cups. It is also considered effective in moving obstructions and so may be used to treat patients in whom a blockage in the circulation of Chi or of blood has been diagnosed.*

USE OF NEEDLES

Despite these various ways of stimulating acupuncture points, the most common form of treatment—and the one that everyone has heard of—is the insertion of needles into the points.

When people who are not familiar with acupuncture therapy hear about needles being stuck into patients, they invariably think of hypodermic needles, injections, and, consequently, pain. Because of this they are

---

*I have heard it said that the suction produced by cupping can be strong enough to cause a sebaceous cyst to burst, drawing out all the cheesy matter contained in it. However, it is not a good idea to allow this to happen. It will remove the cyst temporarily, of course, but the unfortunate thing about sebaceous cysts is that the cheesy matter is contained within a capsule and, unless this capsule is removed, the cyst will re-form. Since cupping is unable to remove the capsule (which can only be done surgically), the cyst is bound to recur. Not only this, but the breaking of its capsule by cupping (or by any other means) can cause inflammation, which can result in the capsule adhering to the surrounding tissues. This is likely to make its removal by surgery more difficult should you ever wish to have it taken out. If you have a sebaceous cyst, therefore, and you suspect that your acupuncturist is going to use cupping, ask him to avoid putting a cup over the cyst itself. Of course, treatment with acupuncture may result in a cyst gradually disappearing; it should certainly help prevent any new cysts from forming.

often unable to understand how acupuncture can so frequently be quite painless. But there are two main reasons why injections are painful, and neither applies to acupuncture.

First, because a fluid has to be passed down a hypodermic needle, the needle is hollow. As it enters the skin, it cuts out a tiny section and pushes it deeper into the tissues, causing pain. Second, the fluid is subsequently injected into the tissues, and because there is no natural cavity there to receive it, it compresses the tissue cells and nerve endings. This too is painful. An acupuncture needle, on the other hand, is very fine. It is not hollow, nor is anything forced down it. Thus its insertion feels quite unlike an injection.

Acupuncture needles come in lengths ranging from one to three inches, and each has a handle that is another inch or two long. At first glance, they may look fairly alarming. However, a needle is rarely inserted to its full length. In areas where there is just a thin layer of flesh overlying a bone, such as the forehead or the hands, only the tip of the needle is inserted; deep insertion is only used in areas of thick muscle, such as the buttocks and thighs.

The length of time that a needle is left in the patient depends on the practitioner and on the treatment being given. Sometimes it is only appropriate to leave a needle in for a second or two. It may be that the purpose is just to puncture the skin and draw off a drop of blood, creating a passageway through which the body can rid itself of invasive Chi. One practitioner I knew, who also practiced manipulation, often inserted a needle briefly into a few points around the area that he intended to manipulate. This had the effect of loosening the surrounding muscles, making the manipulation easier and therefore more comfortable for the patient.

Some practitioners will attach needles to a machine that stimulates them with a mild electrical impulse, causing them to vibrate slightly and producing a mild buzzing sensation. With or without this stimulation, needles may be left in for a period of ten minutes or more. Once they have been inserted, however, the patient usually feels relaxed and comfortable and doesn't find the treatment in any way unpleasant. In fact, in the hands of an expert, patients have been known to feel so relaxed that they have dozed off.

Patients may notice that, at different times, the acupuncturist uses different techniques to insert and remove the needles. This is done according to whether the aim of the treatment is to stimulate the flow of Chi (in a case of deficiency) or to sedate it (in a case of excess). In the former example the acupuncturist might ask the patient to breathe out as he inserts the needle and to breathe in as he takes it out; having extracted it, he may massage the acupuncture point into which it was inserted.

With a patient suffering from an excess of Chi, the needle might be inserted on an inhalation and removed on an exhalation; it might also be rotated while in place. A needle whose function is to stimulate Chi may be inserted so that it lies in the direction of flow of Chi along the meridian, while one intended to reduce Chi might face in the opposite direction.

EAR ACUPUNCTURE

Some needles are designed to remain in position semipermanently. These are the ear studs that are commonly used to help patients who wish to stop smoking or to lose weight. Ear acupuncture was developed in France fairly recently, but it has become very popular, particularly with smokers who are desperate to quit. It is based on the idea that the human body is reflected, in microcosm, in three parts of itself: the hand, the foot, and the ear. Any part of the body can therefore be treated through the corresponding part of the hand, foot, or ear. (This is also the basis of another complementary therapy, reflexology, in which the therapist massages the patient's feet or hands, identifying problems by finding areas of tenderness and treating them by massaging the appropriate points.)

In acupuncture the ear is used in preference to the hand or the foot, but the principle is much the same. A tender area in the ear (as is true anywhere on the body) suggests that the point needs to be treated, and also implies an underlying disorder in the part of the body associated with that point.

So for a patient suffering from, say, a sprained ankle, where there is no long-standing disruption of Chi involved, inserting a single needle in the ear's ankle point may be an appropriate form of treatment. Ear acupuncture is especially useful in the treatment of small children or of patients who are squeamish about needles: inserting a single needle in a place where they cannot see it will cause a minimum of distress.

When using the ear for the treatment of physical disorders there is no need to leave the needles in for longer than the normal period. However, patients who are trying to give up smoking or to diet need continuous help; for them, studs are used that can be left in for about two weeks at a time. These studs are made of a twist of stainless steel and look very much like tiny thumbtacks. If a smoker is being treated, a stud is inserted into the lung point in the ear. For a dieter, a point in the center of the area related to the digestive tract is used. The stud is held in by a Band-Aid. Inserting one may be slightly painful, since the ear is not a very fleshy area, but this pain should only be temporary; after the first hour or so the patient should be perfectly comfortable. Because they are held in by tape, ear studs are not suitable for patients who are allergic to the adhesive on bandages or for those few patients who develop dermatitis when in prolonged contact with metal. I have known allergic patients, however, who were so desperate to give up smoking that they took a course of antihistamine tablets for the period of time that they needed the stud! A better way to do this is perhaps to undergo a course of acupuncture to help resolve the allergies before going on to have an ear stud put in.

Studs are a form of self-help. Every time the patient has a craving for a cigarette (or, in the case of a dieter, every time he starts to get hungry), he gently massages the stud with his finger for about ten or twenty seconds until the craving, or hunger, disappears. Western medicine, which likes to find an empirical reason for everything, has discovered that massage of the stud causes the body to release substances called endorphins into the bloodstream. These naturally occurring painkillers have an effect not dissimilar to that of morphine (hence the name). They probably do play a role in the action of the stud, but their release is unlikely to be the whole story: it does not explain why studs will not work unless they are in exactly the right place, nor why a stud in the lung point will not help a dieter or one in the digestive tract area a smoker.

Of course, a stud will only reduce the *physical* craving or hunger pangs experienced by the patient. A mental desire to smoke or to eat cannot be inhibited by a stud, so the patient must really want to give up smoking or lose weight. It may sound as though it is just a question of mind over matter. Still, there is no doubt that some patients find acupuncture studs to work even when they have had no success with plain willpower or with other treatments—including hypnotherapy, which is unquestionably a mind-over-matter treatment.

The great advantage of acupuncture studs is that they have no side effects. Unlike nicotine chewing gum and appetite suppressants, no drug is entering the patient's system, so studs can continue to be used for as long as it takes the patient to achieve his goal. I knew one woman with a great deal of weight to lose who used a stud for more than eighteen months, during which time she lost a steady two to three pounds a week—something she had never been able to do before.

Although the treatment is perfectly safe for long-term use, the stud itself must be changed about every two weeks. This is because, even though the studs are sterile and made of stainless steel—and often smeared with a little antibiotic cream before insertion—if they stay in over longer periods of time they may act as a focus for infection. To avoid this risk, studs need to be changed regularly. The ear used is alternated to reduce the risk still more. Patients are warned that if the stud becomes painful at any time, they should take it out by simply removing the Band-Aid, which will cause the stud to fall out. (This point should also be remembered by patients who want to wash their hair, take showers, or even go swimming with studs in their ears.)

7

How Acupuncture Works: Patients and Case Histories

To those people who are used to the Western tradition of medicine, the Chinese diagnosis of illness in terms of invasion of the body by wind, heat, or other factors may seem bizarre. You must remember, however, that this diagnosis is intended to be less a literal description of what is going on within the body (although it can sometimes be extremely accurate) than an indication of what form the treatment should take, since diagnosis and treatment are inextricably linked. When an acupuncturist puts a needle into a point that is specific for dispelling wind from the body, he doesn't expect a rush of air to occur, as though it was being released from a pricked balloon. What he does expect, however, is that when he has diagnosed a disease as being due to invasion by wind, the use of such wind-dispelling points will enable him to improve the patient's condition.

ACUPUNCTURE TREATMENT PROTOCOLS

In Western medicine a single diagnosis does not necessarily mean that only one form of treatment is available to the patient. For example, a woman who has abnormally heavy periods may be treated with hormone tablets or with a "scrape" of the uterus. A patient suffering from depression may be offered antidepressant tablets, electroconvulsive therapy, or psychotherapy.

And if a condition is treated with medication, the doctor may be able to choose from among a large number of drugs that work in different ways. But in acupuncture treatment is far more clear-cut. If a patient has a disease that has been caused by invasion by heat, then the treatment is to rid him of the excessive heat, to balance out any consequent imbalance of yin and yang, and to restore the flow of Chi to normal.

For a patient in whom an injury has caused a blockage of the normal flow of Chi (for example, a patient with a sprained ankle) and where pain is being caused by the blockage or by stagnant blood, the treatment is to release the block or disperse the blood. Naturally, this all sounds very unscientific, as well it might when you remember that these are the descriptions that have been used for more than two thousand years. However, it is the indication that these descriptions give us as to treatment that is important. And since in the hands of an expert a diagnosis—and the treatment that automatically follows from it—can produce remarkably beneficial results, it seems unimportant that the diagnosis is couched in terms that have no relevance to modern Western medicine.

In this chapter I want to look at some disorders that are commonly seen in Western medical practice and to consider how an acupuncturist might diagnose and treat them. In each case points will be listed that the acupuncturist might use. However, it is important to note that these are not the only points that might be used, and that of those suitable it is unlikely that more than three or four would be used at one time. In addition, keep in mind that the exact location of the points will vary slightly from individual to individual. The *li*, or *cun* as it is usually called nowadays, is a unit of measurement that may be used to locate acupuncture points. The length of the cun differs from person to person, because it is based upon bodily proportions. For example, the breadth of the four fingers held lightly together is 3 cun and the length of the forearm between the anterior elbow crease and the wrist crease is 12 cun.

Since in real life things are seldom as simple as they seem to be in textbooks, I will also include, at the end, some real case histories in which the points mentioned are those the practitioner actually used.

ARTHRITIS

Since acupuncture is usually associated in people's minds with the idea of pain relief, arthritis is probably one of the most common complaints for which patients initially see an acupuncturist.

Western medicine classifies the majority of arthritis cases as either osteoarthritis or rheumatoid arthritis. Osteoarthritis is a disease that results from wear and tear, and it therefore occurs more commonly in older patients. In younger people it usually develops in joints that have previously been damaged (for example, by a sports injury). It affects the large joints, particularly the hip, which has spent a lifetime carrying the body around. After a joint's natural surfaces have been worn away, deposits of calcium are laid down in it, and the patient finds that the joint becomes stiff and causes pain, especially upon movement. Rheumatoid arthritis, on the other hand, is an inflammatory condition that can affect people of any age, including children (when it is known as Still's disease). On the whole, it attacks the smaller joints, which become inflamed and distorted. Some patients recover completely while others may be left crippled, but the majority of people who suffer from rheumatoid arthritis experience a certain degree of disability without it ever becoming severe. For some reason this condition is much more common in women than men.

The main feature of both types of arthritis is that the joints are painful and stiff and may be swollen. Chinese diagnosis ascribes these symptoms to a blockage to the flow of Chi, either because the meridians affected have been invaded by external harmful Chi or because a meridian has been damaged by injury.

Damage to a meridian may at first remain quite localized, but if it is untreated, the disruption to the flow of Chi may spread and affect other meridians. For example, if a soccer player is kicked on the side of his knee, it can become bruised and swollen. This may then resolve so that his knee returns to normal. On the other hand, if he tries to play soccer while the joint is still recovering, this could interfere with healing and the condition could become chronic. A Western physician would say that the initial blow has set up a reaction within the joint that, aggravated by further stress, has resulted in the development of an arthritic condition. A Chinese physician might say that the initial blow disrupted the flow of Chi in the Gall Bladder meridian, which runs down the side of the knee; because the flow was not allowed to return to normal, the disruption has spread to involve the Urinary Bladder meridian running down the back of the leg, the Stomach meridian running down the front of the leg, and then the Liver, Kidney, and Spleen meridians. Ultimately there was a circle around the knee through which the flow of Chi was blocked.

It is the blockage of Chi that causes the pain and the swelling. The acupuncturist's treatment will attempt to relieve the block and disperse any invasive Chi that may have been the precipitating cause. However, arthritis often occurs in more than just one joint, and our athlete is not the typical arthritic patient.

Let us take the imaginary case of a middle-aged woman who comes to see the acupuncturist complaining of pain in her joints. She has had this for some years and it has gradually been getting worse. It is particularly bad if the weather is wet or cold but, to some extent, it is relieved by warmth; she finds that she is more mobile in the summer months. The pain in her wrists and the numbness and pain in her fingers make it increasingly difficult for her to do housework, sew, or write a letter.

Two important points in this history are that the condition is chronic and that it is made worse by cold and damp. It would seem, therefore, that cold and damp may be the external factors involved (since both of these tend to produce chronic conditions). Conditions that present with painful joints (including those that in the West are diagnosed as arthritis, rheumatic fever, and gout) are commonly known in Chinese medicine as bi syndromes. *Bi* implies an obstruction—both to the flow of Chi and to the blood. This woman would seem to have a bi syndrome caused by an invasion by cold and damp.

Upon examination this patient is found to have some swelling around the affected joints. This too suggests an obstruction to the flow of Chi. Her tongue has a thin, moist, white coating—which, in a patient who is unwell, suggests an invasion by cold and damp. Finally, her pulse is deep and slow. This indicates that the condition is internal—and therefore chronic—and cold in nature.

To treat this patient, the acupuncturist would use points that disperse the invading cold and damp and remove the obstruction to the flow of Chi. Because of the chronicity of the condition, the body's production of protective Chi also needs to be stimulated, to help the patient fight back. And the acupuncturist might also treat specific areas, such as the wrists and hands, that are particularly troublesome. Moxibustion, with its effect of warming the acupuncture points, would be particularly useful in counteracting the invasive cold and damp. Table 1 shows some of the points that might be used.

The overall effect of treatment will be to unblock obstructed meridians, clear out invading cold and damp, and stimulate the circulation of blood and Chi around the body. Of course, it may happen that the patient's hands and wrists are too painful to withstand the insertion of needles on the first visit. In this case the acupuncturist will use the points located farther away from the painful areas and will begin to use the local points only as the patient's condition improves.

Now let us look at a patient who, in Western terms, has had an acute attack of rheumatoid arthritis. The interesting thing here is that both this patient and the middle-aged woman just described might be treated by a Western practitioner with the same sorts of drugs—painkillers, anti-inflammatory preparations, or possibly even steroids. To an acupuncturist, however, the two patients are treated quite differently from each other, because they are diagnosed as suffering from different conditions.

Let us assume that this second patient is a thirty-year-old woman who has recently developed swelling and pain in several of her joints. She has a mild fever, and the affected joints are red and feel hot to the touch. The pain in her joints is not constant, as it was with the older woman; some days her knees are the most painful, on other days it is her wrists, and sometimes her feet are most troublesome.

TABLE I. OSTEOARTHRITIS TREATMENT

Point	Name	Meaning	Location	Function
LI 4	Hegu	Valley Junction	On the back of the hand, in the angle between the thumb and forefinger	Dispels cold; clears obstructed Chi; relieves pain and weakness in the hands and arms
LI 5	Yangxi	Stream of Yang	On the side of the wrist, above the thumb	Used for its local effects on the hand and wrist
St 36	Zusanli	Three Li on Lower Limbs	Three Li below the knee	Relieves stiffness in joints by nourishing the tendons and muscles
Sp 10	Xuehai	Sea of Blood	On the inside of the leg, just above the bend of the knee	Tonifies Chi and promotes its circulation; also stimulates blood; moxibustion can be used to disperse damp and cold
SI 4	Wangu	Wrist bone	On the side of the wrist, above the little finger	Relieves pain in the arm and fingers and weakness of the wrist
SJ 3	Zhong-zhu	Land in the Middle of Water	On the back of the hand, surrounded by other points	Has specific action on the hands
SJ 4	Yangchi	Pool of Yang	On the back of the wrist	Stimulates the flow of Chi and removes obstructions; also used for its local effects on the hand and wrist
SJ 5	Waiguan	Lateral Pass	A short distance above SJ 4 on the lateral side of the humerus bone	Acts in the same way as SJ 4
SJ 6	Zhigou	Ditch of the Limb	A little way above the wrist, on the back of the forearm, in the "ditch" between the radius and ulna bones	Stimulates the flow of Chi; clears stagnation
Ren 6	Qihai	Sea of Chi	On the abdomen, on the midline, a little way below the umbilicus	Tonifies Chi and promotes its circulation

Listening to her story, the acupuncturist decides that there has been an invasion by heat (causing the redness of the joints and the fever) and by wind (causing the pain to flit from one joint to another). Looking at her, he sees that her face is flushed, indicating the presence of a hot disease. Her tongue is red and has a yellow coating, and her pulse is rapid and forceful; all this confirms the diagnosis of an invasion by heat.

Some of the points the acupuncturist might use to treat rheumatoid

TABLE 2. RHEUMATOID ARTHRITIS TREATMENT

Point	Name	Meaning	Location	Function
LI 11	Quchi	Crooked Pool	In a depression at the lateral side of the elbow crease	Eliminates heat and wind; used for its local effects on the wrist; reduces pain and swelling in joints
LI 15	Jianyu	Corner of Shoulder	Just below the point of the shoulder	Eliminates heat and wind; disperses stagnant Chi
St 45	Lidui	Door of the Stomach	At the end of the meridian on the second toe, just behind the corner of the nail	Eliminates wind; has a specific action on the knees and feet
UB 12	Fengmen	Gate of the Wind	To the side of the vertebral column, approximately level with the upper point of the shoulder blade, at a point where the body is easily invaded by wind	Specific for arthritic conditions, particularly when caused by wind
SJ 5	Waiguan	Lateral Pass	Just above the wrist on the lateral side of the humerus bone	Eliminates heat; local point for treating the wrist

arthritis are shown in table 2. Here again, the overall effect of treatment is to dispel the causative factors—in this case, wind and heat—and to unblock obstructions to the flow of Chi. Once Chi is flowing normally again and the heat and wind have been dispersed, the patient's joints will be able to return to normal.

MIGRAINE

This is another complaint that often finds its way into the acupuncturist's clinic, since Western medicine cannot always treat it successfully.

A commonly held medical theory of migraine is that it is caused by an abnormal spasm, followed by an abnormal dilation, of the arteries in the brain, specifically those supplying its front part. The initial spasm results in insufficient blood flowing to the eyes, which is why many patients experience visual symptoms—flashing lights or even total blindness—at the start of a migraine. Then the arteries relax and dilate, and an abnormally large amount of blood flows into the area that was so recently deprived. It is this great surge of blood that causes the severe headache. Once the migraine has developed, ordinary painkillers such as aspirin and acetaminophen usually have little effect on it. The aim of Western medical treatment is to stop the migraine before it gets to this stage by preventing the arteries from behaving in this abnormal way. The ergot derivatives that form the basis of a number of migraine treatments are vasoconstrictors—they prevent overdilation of the arteries and so stop the headache from developing.

Let us now look at a young woman who comes to the acupuncture clinic complaining of recurrent migraine. She describes the pain that she experiences during an attack as running from just above one eye across the top of her head and down into her neck. It is severe and throbbing, and her face becomes hot and flushed.

And let us say that, on her way to her appointment, the patient starts to develop a migraine; by the time she sees the acupuncturist, the headache is becoming quite severe. Looking at her, the acupuncturist sees that her face is red, indicating a hot condition. When he examines her eyes, they appear inflamed, and she complains that the light hurts them. This suggests that the heat is a result of an excess of yang. Her tongue is red and has a yellow coating, which again signifies heat. Her pulse is rapid due to the heat, and is both forceful and floating in character, indicating an external syndrome with an excess of yang.

The treatment of this patient, therefore, would be aimed at reducing this overabundance of yang and bringing yin and yang back into balance. This will then cool the heat that has arisen as a result of excessive yang. The path that the pain takes—from the eye across the head and into the neck—corresponds to the route of the Gall Bladder meridian in this part of the body, a meridian that is often disturbed in patients with migraine. The acupuncturist may feel along the course of the meridian for tender points that need treatment. One acupuncture teacher I knew called them, rather accurately, "ouch points," but their Chinese name is *ah-shi* (meaning "oh, yes!") points. If the patient has been suffering from recurrent migraine, these points will probably be tender even between attacks.

Treatment can either be given during the migraine itself, to stop the attack, or between migraines when the patient feels well. In either case the balancing out of yin and yang should help prevent further attacks. The patient may also be advised to stop smoking, drinking alcohol, and eating red meats, since these are factors that can stimulate the formation of excess yang.

Table 3 shows some of the points that might be used in the treatment of this patient.

TABLE 3. MIGRAINE TREATMENT

Point	Name	Meaning	Location	Function
St 8	Touwei	Angle of the Head	At the corner of the forehead, just within the hairline	A specific point for the treatment of migraine
SJ 5	Waiguan	Lateral Pass	Just above the wrist on the lateral side of the humerus bone	An important point for treating external conditions, clearing heat, and restoring yang to normal
GB 14	Yangbai	Yang Brightness	A little way above the midpoint of the eyebrow	May be an ah-shi point in this condition; brightens the eyes (hence the name)
GB 17	Zhengying	Fright and Fear	Just lateral to the crown of the head	May be an ah-shi point in this condition; can treat fright and fear (hence the name)
GB 20	Fengchi	Wind Pool	At the back of the neck, in the depression below the base of the skull	May be an ah-shi point in this condition; an important point for eliminating wind
GB 41	Zu-linqui	Foot-Treating Tears	On the lateral side of the foot	Indicated in the treatment of several eye conditions

ASTHMA AND BRONCHITIS

These two conditions can be either acute or chronic, and they can affect people of any age. Western medicine has little to offer in the way of cure once they have become chronic, although it can often control them very effectively through the use of drugs. However, many people do not like the idea of having to take drugs for the rest of their lives, and some start to look for an alternative form of therapy.

Asthma is often considered by Western practitioners to be an allergic phenomenon in which the bronchi, or tubes, of the lung constrict and so impede the flow of air into and out of the lung. It is becoming increasingly prevalent, especially in young people, perhaps as a result of air pollution. In many people it is caused by an allergy to pollen, and an attack of hay fever may lead into an attack of asthma. In other cases children who have had eczema (another allergic problem) when young sometimes develop asthma later on, though their skin condition may improve. This would be an indication to an acupuncturist that the disease was turning from an external syndrome into an internal one. Treatment might well result in a return of the eczema before the patient's recovery is complete.

In many cases of allergic asthma, the allergen (the substance to which the patient is allergic) is house dust. Other common allergens are feathers and animal fur, so birds, cats, dogs, and horses will set off an attack if they come near the patient. Asthma also has a psychological component: Because it is a very frightening condition, the fear that arises when an attack starts may itself make the attack worse, forming a vicious circle.

Asthma may be associated with bronchitis in an individual patient, but the two conditions can occur independently of each other. Bronchitis is an inflammatory condition of the bronchi brought on by anything that causes the lung to become inflamed, such as infection or smoking. An acute attack, which presents as a bad cough accompanied by the production of large amounts of yellow or green phlegm, and which is due to a bacterial infection, may be completely cured by treatment with antibiotics. However, a series of attacks can cause permanent damage to the lung, especially if the attacks are inadequately treated, there is another contributory condition such as asthma present, or the patient is a smoker, which will prevent the bronchitis from ever resolving completely. If this is the case, the patient may go on to develop chronic bronchitis, with a permanent productive cough and shortness of breath—a condition commonly seen in patients who have smoked heavily for years.

Let us take as an example, first of all, a patient who would be diagnosed by a Western physician as having asthma. He is a young man who periodically develops a tight feeling in his chest that makes it difficult for him to breathe. During these attacks he wheezes and coughs up some white frothy sputum. If he gets upset, this may bring on an attack. Upon examination he is found to have a sticky white coating on his tongue and a slow pulse that feels like a taut wire. From these symptoms and signs, the acupuncturist can diagnose that the patient has congestion in his lungs attributable to invasion by cold (because the pulse is slow) and by phlegm (because of the sputum and the appearance of the tongue). The bowstring pulse indicates that the congestion is secondary to spasm, which is preventing the normal flow of Chi. This type of asthma is also said to be brought on by exposure to a cold wind when the patient is tired, and it may be made worse by emotion.

Treatment of this patient by a Western physician would use drugs to relax the spasms in the bronchi. An acupuncturist, on the other hand, would select points to disperse the cold and the phlegm, and use moxa or cupping to warm the lung. Some of the points that might be used are shown in table 4.

Our second hypothetical patient is somewhat older than the first—in his fifties—but presents with the same tight feeling in his chest and wheezy breathing. In addition, he has a slight fever and a chesty cough. The spasms in his chest prevent him from coughing up very much sputum, but what does come up is thick and either yellow or green. Upon examination his pulse is fast and slippery or gliding in quality. His tongue is red and has a sticky yellow coating. The diagnosis here

TABLE 4. COLD-INDUCED ASTHMA TREATMENT

Point	Name	Meaning	Location	Function
Lu 7	Lieque	Broken Clouds	On the thumb side of the wrist, above the bony prominence	Activates lung Chi
Lu 9	Taiyuan	Great Abundant Pool	On the wrist above the thumb, at a point where the Chi of the meridian is abundant	Disperses phlegm
St 40	Fenlong	Great Abundance	On the side of the leg, at the lowest part of the calf, at a point where Chi flows abundantly	Disperses phlegm
UB 12	Fengmen	Gate of the Wind	To the side of the vertebral column, approximately level with the upper point of the shoulder blade	Eliminates cold; has a specific effect in the treament of asthma
Ren 17	Shanzhong	Middle Exposure	In the exposed central part of the chest, along the midline between the nipples	Strengthens the Chi of the lung; has a specific effect in the treatment of asthma
Ren 22	Tiantu	Chimney of Heaven	In the midline depression at the base of the neck, above the breastbone, where the windpipe acts as a chimney for the Chi of the lung	An important local point for the treatment of respiratory diseases; has a specific effect in the treatment of asthma

is one of invasion of the lung by heat, which has caused stagnation of Chi and the formation of phlegm. This is indicated by the fever, fast pulse, and red tongue with yellow coating, all of which signify heat; the slippery pulse, sputum, and stickiness of the tongue coating all point to the presence of phlegm.

A Western doctor would prescribe a bronchorelaxant drug and an antibiotic. An acupuncturist could choose from among a number of points, some of which are shown in table 5 (page 126).

Still on the topic of asthma, let us finally look at a child who has chronic asthma and whom a Western physician would treat in a similar way to the two patients already mentioned. This little boy, let us say, is eight years

TABLE 5. HEAT-INDUCED ASTHMA TREATMENT

Point	Name	Meaning	Location	Function
Lu 5	Chize	Ulnar Marsh	In a depression next to the ulna bone, in the crease of the elbow	Clears heat from the lung; alleviates stagnation; an important point of regulating the Chi of the lung
St 40	Fenlong	Great Abundance	On the lateral side of the leg at the lowest part of the calf, a point where Chi flows abundantly	Disperses phlegm
UB 13	Feishu	Lung shu point	To the side of the spine, near the upper border of the shoulder blade	Strengthens the Chi of the lung
Ren 22	Tiantu	Chimney of Heaven	In the midline depression at the base of the neck, above the breastbone, where the windpipe acts as a chimney for the Chi of the lung	Stimulates the circulation of Chi in the lung; is a special point for the treatment of asthma

old and has had asthma since the age of three. The recurrent attacks have interfered with his normal development, and he is underweight and short for his age. He gets tired easily and is inclined to be restless. Upon examination his face has a yellowish tinge, and his lips are pale. His tongue looks pale and has a thin, white, sticky coating; his pulse feels forceless and disappears upon pressure. The characteristics of his pulse along with the color of his face and lips suggest that this is a xu, or deficiency, condition. This is also suggested by the fact that the boy is small and underweight. His pale tongue, too, indicates a deficiency, while its sticky white coating points to an invasion by cold and damp or phlegm. The deficiency has obviously affected the lung, producing the symptoms of asthma, but since the kidney is the organ in charge of growth and development, there would seem to be a deficiency there as well. According to the Law of the Five Elements, the Lung meridian, which is metal, is mother to the Kidney meridian—which is, of course, water. So a long-term deficiency in one can easily affect the other.

One possible treatment for this patient is shown in table 6. Obviously, a long-term problem such as his would need an extended course of treat-

TABLE 6. CHRONIC ASTHMA TREATMENT FOR A CHILD

Point	Name	Meaning	Location	Function
Lu 9	Taiyuan	Great Abundant Pool	On the wrist above the thumb, at a point where the Chi of the meridian is abundant	Forms a direct link with the lung and can be used to stimulate it; as Earth point of the Lung meridian, it can be used in accordance with the Law of the Five Elements*
UB 13	Feishu	Lung shu point	To the side of the spine, near the upper border of the shoulder blade	Removes blockages in the lung; stimulates the circulation of Chi
UB 23	Shenshu	Kidney shu point	To the side of the spine, at about the level of the waist	Stimulates the functional Chi of the kidney
K 3	Taixi	Great Canyon	On the medial side of the ankle, in the depression beside the Achilles tendon	Stimulates the functional Chi of the kidney
Du 4	Mingmen	Gate of Life	Along the midline of the back at the level of the kidney, whose Chi is the basic source for the whole body	Stimulates the functional Chi of the kidney

*The Lung is the yin Metal meridian and it is the child of the Spleen meridian, which is the yin Earth meridian. Taiyuan is the Earth point of the Lung meridian and so can be used to stimulate the yin Earth meridian. In this way the mother can be stimulated to nourish the child. (See chapter 3.)

ment. The points used would probably vary from session to session, too, depending on how his condition was reacting.

I have already noted that asthma and bronchitis can exist independently, so finally in this section let us bring into our imaginary acupuncture clinic two patients suffering from bronchitis—one with the acute condition, the other with the chronic.

Let us say that the first of these patients became ill a week or so ago, when he developed a head cold with a runny nose, fever, and general feeling of being unwell. Since then he has started to cough and is bringing up quantities of thick yellow sputum. Such complaints are of course regularly seen in general practitioners' offices during the winter months, and they are usually treated with a course of antibiotics. Upon examining the patient the acupuncturist finds that he has a rapid pulse, a flushed face, and a red tongue with a thin yellow coating. All this points to a diagnosis of an invasion by heat; the thin yellow coating on the tongue suggests that wind may also be involved. If wind invades the lung and blocks the circulation of Chi, phlegm will form, and the fact that the patient has been coughing up sputum is another indication that this is what has happened.

Table 7 shows some of the points that might be used in treating this patient.

The treatment of the patient with chronic bronchitis is somewhat different. He complains of a constant cough that becomes worse in winter, along with a lack of appetite and energy. Western medicine applies the

TABLE 7. ACUTE BRONCHITIS TREATMENT

Point	Name	Meaning	Location	Function
Lu 7	Lieque	Broken Clouds	Above the bony prominence on the thumb side of the wrist	Strengthens the Chi of the lung
LI 4	Hegu	Valley Junction	On the back of the hand, in the angle between the thumb and forefinger	An important point for treating diseases of the lung because both the Large Intestine and Lung are Metal meridians; eliminates heat and relieves obstruction of Chi
LI 11	Quchi	Crooked Pool	In a depression at the lateral side of the elbow crease	Expels wind
St 40	Fenlong	Great Abundance	On the lateral side of the leg, at the lowest part of the calf, at a point where Chi flows abundantly	Eliminates phlegm
UB 12	Fengmen	Gate of the Wind	To the side of the vertebral column, approximately level with the upper point of the shoulder blade	Expels wind
UB 13	Feishu	Lung shu point	To the side of the spine, near the upper border of the shoulder blade	Strengthens the Chi of the lung

term *bronchitis* to him as well as to the last patient, because both are seen as having an inflammation (*-itis*) of the tubes of the lung. However, Chinese medicine always emphasizes the fundamental difference between acute and chronic conditions: *Acute* implies external and often hot syndromes, possibly with an excess of yang, while *chronic* suggests internal, cold, and excessively yin syndromes. When the acupuncturist examines the chronic bronchitic patient, he finds a pale tongue and a deep, slow pulse. These, together with his symptoms of flagging appetite and energy, suggest a xu (deficiency) syndrome. The patient's tongue has a sticky white coating, which indicates that cold and damp or phlegm are factors in the causation of the disease. So treatment would be aimed at stimulating the energy of the lungs and dispelling the cold and phlegm.

Table 8 shows the points that might be used to treat this patient.

Naturally, a patient with chronic bronchitis will need a much longer course of treatment than one with acute bronchitis in order to obtain relief from his symptoms.

TABLE 8. CHRONIC BRONCHITIS TREATMENT

Point	Name	Meaning	Location	Function
Lu 9	Taiyuan	Great Abundant Pool	On the wrist above the thumb, at a point where the Chi of the meridian is abundant	Stimulates the Earth meridians, encouraging the Spleen meridian to nourish its child, the Lung meridian*
UB 20	Pishu	Spleen shu point	To the side of the spine, above the level of the waist and below the shoulder blade	Acts in the same way as Lu 9*
UB 23	Shenshu	Kidney shu point	To the side of the spine, at about the level of the waist	Stimulates the kidney to prevent any deficiency in that meridian contributing to the deficiency in the lung[†]
K 3	Taixi	Great Canyon	On the medial aspect of the ankle, in the depression beside the Achilles tendon	Acts in the same way as UB 23[†]

*The spleen is responsible for the transport and transformation of the nutrients that form Chi. If it malfunctions, retention of water in the body can result. This may materialize in the lung as phlegm.
†Because the Kidney meridian is the yin Water meridian and therefore the child of the Lung meridian, UB 23 and K 3 are used to stimulate the kidney. (See chapter 3.)

GALLBLADDER DISEASE

This is not a problem you might immediately think of taking to an acupuncturist for treatment, since in Western practice it is usually dealt with surgically. Western physicians divide it into two main types: cholecystitis (inflammation of the gallbladder) and cholelithiasis (gallstones). Very often the two occur together. Both are painful conditions and commonly occur in women around the age of forty; the patients are frequently overweight. Cholecystitis often has an acute onset, with the patient complaining of a constant severe pain just under the base of the rib cage on the right-hand side, sometimes accompanied by fever and vomiting. Usually the cause is an infection, sometimes due to the fact that there are stones in the gallbladder, and Western treatment might consist of antibiotics in the acute stage followed by removal of the gallbladder later on when the infection has settled down. When uncomplicated by infection, gallstones are more likely to be associated with a colicky, or spasmodic, pain due to the gallbladder trying to squeeze the stone out or to a stone actually passing down the bile duct leading from the gallbladder to the small intestine. In either condition jaundice may occur if the flow of bile into the small intestine is blocked either by the inflammation or by a stone. Because the symptoms of the two complaints may be very similar, it may be necessary to take Xrays to establish whether or not gallstones are present. A gallbladder that contains stones, whether or not it is causing symptoms, is usually removed complete with stones.

In order to see how such a patient might be treated by acupuncture, let us imagine that an acupuncturist is called to see a thirty-nine-year-old woman who is complaining of a severe pain under the right side of her rib cage, along with fever and jaundice. Upon examination her tongue is found to be red with a sticky yellow coating; her pulse is rapid and forceful. The location of the pain indicates a problem with the liver and gallbladder, which lie together under the right-hand border of the rib cage. Jaundice is usually seen as an indication of invasion by damp heat. This is corroborated by the appearance of the patient's tongue and her fever. The forceful quality of her pulse suggests a shi (excess) syndrome, and the involvement of heat further suggests that it is yang that is in excess.

Some points that the acupuncturist might use are shown in table 9.

TABLE 9. GALLBLADDER DISEASE TREATMENT

Point	Name	Meaning	Location	Function
UB 18	Ganshu	Liver shu point	Lateral to the spine, between the levels of the waist and the armpit	Stimulates Chi; relieves obstruction
UB 19	Danshu	Gall Bladder shu point	Just below UB 18	Stimulates Chi; relieves obstruction
GB 34	Yangling-quan	Yang Mound Spring	In a depression below the bony prominence on the lateral aspect of the knee	Stimulates Chi; relieves obstruction
Liv 2	Xingjian	Walking Between	Between the first and second toes	Reduces heat in the liver; mobilizes Chi that has become stuck*
Liv 3	Taichong	Great Pass	On the upper aspect of the foot, along a line that runs between the first and second toes	Clears away heat; suppresses excess yang
Ren 12	Zhong-wan	Middle of Stomach	Along the midline of the abdomen, a little way above the umbilicus	Expels damp and heat

*Liv 2 is also the Fire point of the meridian. Fire is the child of wood, and the Liver and Gall Bladder are Wood meridians. In a shi syndrome it is customary to treat the child, while in a xu syndrome you treat the mother. (See chapter 3.)

HYPERTENSION (HIGH BLOOD PRESSURE)

Although modern drugs can control hypertension very effectively in the majority of cases, they may cause side effects. In addition, it is usually necessary for the patient to continue to take the tablets for the rest of his life. A therapy such as acupuncture, which does not have these drawbacks, may therefore seem attractive.

Western medicine cannot fully explain the cause of most cases of hypertension, which are lumped together under the name *idiopathic*—in other words, "cause unknown." That it is associated with atheroma (hardening of the arteries), heart disease, and strokes is firmly established, but there is still some confusion as to what comes first: Does the atheroma cause the hypertension or is it the other way around? The presence of one is likely to worsen the other and so create a vicious circle.

Hypertension often produces no symptoms in its early stages and is picked up only when the patient has his blood pressure checked during a routine medical examination. As we have seen, however, diagnoses in Chinese medicine are based upon the patient's symptoms and outward signs, backed up by pulse and tongue observations. Elevated blood pressure is not recognized per se in traditional Chinese medicine because, naturally, when acupuncture was first developing thousands of years ago, there was no equipment for measuring blood pressure. However, if a patient whose blood pressure has been found to be raised upon testing but has no symptoms goes to an acupuncturist, examination of his tongue and pulse (plus the other signs used by practitioners of the Five Elements school) should indicate a diagnosis in Chinese medical terms. And his treatment will then be based on this.

Let us consider, for example, a patient who has already developed symptoms from her hypertension. She is an elderly lady, rather frail, who is complaining of slight dizziness, blurred vision, and recurring headaches. She also has difficulty in sleeping and wakes early in the morning. Her face is pale but she has pink cheeks. Her tongue is red and slightly glossy in appearance, and she has a weak and rapid pulse.

TABLE 10. EXCESSIVE-YANG HYPERTENSION TREATMENT

Point	Name	Meaning	Location	Function
UB 23	Shenshu	Kidney shu point	To the side of the spine, at about the level of the waist	Stimulates the function of the kidney
K 3	Taixi	Great Canyon	On the medial aspect of the ankle, in the depression beside the Achilles tendon	Stimulates the yin and sedates the yang of the liver and kidney
Liv 2	Xingjian	Walking Between	Between the first and second toes	Stimulates yin and sedates yang; usually used with Liv 3 in the control of high blood pressure
Liv 3	Taichong	Great Pass	On the upper aspect of the foot, along a line that runs between the first and second toes	Reduces heat in the liver; usually used with Liv 2 in the control of high blood pressure

Hypertension is said to be due either to an excess of yang or an excess of phlegm and damp. In this woman's case the former would seem to be the cause; it is suggested by her pale face and pink cheeks, which indicate a yin deficiency resulting in a relative excess of yang. Such a deficiency may occur in the liver or kidney (which control the circulation of Chi) simply as a result of growing old. A yin deficiency in the kidney will result in its child, the liver, becoming undernourished. The resulting relative hyperactivity of the liver's yang may produce dizziness. Headaches, a red tongue, and a rapid pulse also indicate an excess of yang (producing an inner heat), while a coexisting deficiency of yin is suggested by the blurred vision, sleeping problems, glossy tongue, and weakness of the pulse. Blurred vision is particularly associated with a deficiency in the liver, which is linked to the eye.

This patient may be helped by treatment using some of the points shown in table 10.

If hypertension is caused by an invasion of phlegm and damp, the picture is quite different. We may imagine in this case a middle-aged man who, like the previous patient, complains of dizziness, but unlike her he is not frail but overweight. He also suffers from palpitations and occasional chest pain. Upon examination he is found to have a slow and deep pulse, and his tongue has a sticky coating. Because it is related to eating habits, obesity is said to have a damaging effect on the spleen, which distills Chi from ingested food. As a result the formation and circulation of Chi is affected. The sticky coating on this patient's tongue suggests that phlegm and damp have developed in conjunction with the poor circulation of Chi. His deep, slow pulse indicates an internal syndrome and corroborates the findings on the tongue.

Retention of phlegm and damp within the body causes mental clouding and would be the reason for this patient's dizziness. His treatment would consist of clearing out the phlegm and thus returning the function of the spleen to normal. Some of the points that might be used are shown in table 11.

TABLE 11. PHLEGM- AND DAMP-INDUCED HYPERTENSION TREATMENT

Point	Name	Meaning	Location	Function
St 40	Fenlong	Great Abundance	On the lateral aspect of the leg at the lowest part of the calf, a point where Chi flows abundantly	Expels phlegm and damp
Liv 2	Xingjian	Walking Between	Between the first and second toes	Mobilizes Chi that has become obstructed
Ren 12	Zhongwan	Middle of Stomach	Along the midline of the abdomen, a little way above the umbilicus	A specific point for treating hypertension

URTICARIA

In Western medicine urticaria (hives) is seen as an allergic problem and often occurs as a reaction to eating things such as shellfish or strawberries. It may also occur as a result of emotional trauma. Its other name is nettle rash because the rash that it produces looks very similar to that which might be seen on someone who has been badly stung by nettles.

If we picture a woman with urticaria, she has large raised red patches on her arms, legs, trunk, and face. These appeared suddenly and are hot and itchy. Upon examination her tongue is red with a thin yellow coating, and her pulse is superficial in character and rapid. The redness of her skin patches, together with her red tongue and rapid pulse, suggest an invasion by heat, while the suddenness of onset and the yellow coating on the tongue indicate that wind is also involved. Treatment will therefore aim at eliminating both of these factors. Table 12 shows some of the points that might be used.

TABLE 12. URTICARIA TREATMENT

Point	Name	Meaning	Location	Function
LI 4	Hegu	Valley Junction	On the back of the hand, in the angle between the thumb and forefinger	Expels heat; is specific for the treatment of skin conditions
LI 11	Quchi	Crooked Pool	In a depression at the lateral side of the elbow crease	Expels wind
Sp 10	Xuehai	Sea of Blood	On the inside of the leg, just above the bend of the knee	Expels heat; simulates the flow of Chi; is often used to treat inflamed skin conditions
UB 17	Geshu	Diaphragm shu point	To the side of the spine, between the level of the armpit and that of the lower border of the shoulder blade	Expels wind by treating the blood and returning its flow to normal

TINNITUS (RINGING IN THE EARS)

This is another fairly common chronic problem but, unfortunately, one for which Western medicine has very little to offer. It can be helped by various complementary therapies, however, including hypnotherapy, homeopathy, and of course acupuncture.

In Western medical terms tinnitus is caused by damage to the nerve that supplies the inner ear; it is therefore usually associated with deafness. The patient's hearing is poor on two counts: first due to the nerve damage and, second, because the tinnitus masks whatever sounds are able to get through. So, if the tinnitus can be diminished, the patient will hear better whether or not the deafness itself has been reduced.

Let us take as our example a patient with what is known in Western terms as Ménière's disease or syndrome, which consists of ringing in the ears, dizziness, and gradually worsening deafness. He is a man in his seventies, and he tells the acupuncturist that his tinnitus becomes worse if he gets upset or stressed. He has a weak pulse, and his tongue looks pale.

I noted above, in connection with the elderly lady with hypertension, that old age may be associated with reduced functioning of the kidney and a reduction in its functional Chi. The sense organ with which the kidney is linked is the ear, so a chronic deficiency of Chi in the elderly may reduce the ear's ability to function normally and thus cause deafness. This patient's deep, weak pulse and his pale tongue, together with the fact that his symptoms are aggravated by stress, all suggest the presence of a xu (deficiency) syndrome. The dizziness is due to a deficiency in the brain (or Sea of Marrow), whose maintenance is dependent on the normal functioning of the kidney.

In treatment the aim is to strengthen the kidney and reinforce its functional Chi. This may be done by using some of the points shown in table 13.

TABLE 13. TINNITUS TREATMENT

Point	Name	Meaning	Location	Function
Sp 6	Sanyinjiao	Three Yin Meridians Crossing	At the intersection point of the Spleen, Liver, and Kidney meridians, on the medial aspect of the leg, a short way above the ankle	Stimulates kidney and liver*
UB 23	Shenshu	Kidney shu point	To the side of the spine, at about the level of the waist	Stimulates kidney Chi
K 3	Taixi	Great Canyon	On the medial aspect of the ankle, in the depression beside the Achilles tendon	Stimulates kidney Chi
GB 2	Tinghui	Gathering of Hearing	Just in front of the ear, at the joint of the jaw	A specific point for treating deafness and tinnitus, due to its position next to the ear
Liv 3	Taichong	Great Pass	On the upper aspect of the foot, along a line that runs between the first and second toes	Reinforces the yin element of the kidney and liver
Du 4	Mingmen	Gate of Life	Along the midline of the back, at the level of the kidney	Strengthens the yang of the kidney

*Here again, the treatment is based on the relationship between the Kidney (Water) and the Liver (Wood) meridians. The former is the mother of the latter, and a deficiency in one will, if long continued, affect the other. (See chapter 3.)

DEPRESSION

This is not the sort of problem you might at first think could be helped by acupuncture. We often tend to associate the use of acupuncture with purely physical problems, and even though there is no doubt that an imbalance of chemicals in the brain can cause clinical depression, it is primarily a mental condition. The truth, however, is that acupuncture can have remarkable effects on mental states: Like many other complementary therapies, it treats the whole patient by raising his entire level of health, increasing his ability to shake off whatever symptoms are troubling him, whether they be physical or mental.

Here we may imagine a middle-aged woman who is complaining of depression that has crept up on her very gradually over the past few months. She also feels very anxious, often without knowing why—a common accompaniment to depression. She has difficulty in sleeping and experiences the early-morning wakefulness typical of clinical depression, awakening at around five in the morning and unable to fall asleep again. She also has occasional bouts of dizziness and feels totally devoid of energy all the time. Upon examination her face is pale, and her skin looks dull. Her tongue appears flabby, and there are indentations around its edge made by her teeth. Her pulse is slow and disappears upon pressure. These findings, together with her symptoms, all point to a deficiency syndrome. Since the heart is the seat of the mind, it would seem that her deficiency of Chi has affected the Heart meridian. Treatment would therefore be aimed at stimulating the production and circulation of Chi and ensuring adequate nourishment of the heart.

Table 14 shows some of the points that might be used for treating this woman.

TABLE 14. DEPRESSION TREATMENT

Point	Name	Meaning	Location	Function
H 3	Shaoha	Young Sea	At the medial end of the elbow crease, where the Chi of the meridian circulates like water flowing	An important point for the treatment of depression, strengthening the heart
H 7	Shenmen	Door of the Mind	Along the crease of the wrist, above the little finger	Strengthens the Chi of the heart
UB 15	Xinshu	Heart shu point	To the side of the spine, a little above the level of the armpit	Strengthens the Chi of the heart
UB 20	Pishu	Spleen shu point	To the side of the spine, above the level of the waist and some way below UB 15	Stimulates the spleen; promotes the absorption and circulation of Chi*
UB 21	Weishu	Stomach shu point	To the side of the spine, above the level of the waist and just below UB 20	Stimulates the stomach; promotes the absorption and circulation of Chi*

*A general lowering of Chi in the body may result from a malfunction of the spleen or stomach, which are responsible for extracting Chi from ingested food.

INSOMNIA

Many people suffer from insomnia at one time or another. Usually it is a temporary problem, often caused by the patient going through a stressful period. If he is prepared to wait, he is likely to find that the problem resolves itself as soon as the stress has passed. However, many patients become so anxious about their inability to sleep that this anxiety itself contributes to the insomnia, turning an acute state into a chronic problem. Such patients may see their doctors and ask for sleeping pills, intending to take them for just a week or two until they are sleeping normally again. Unfortunately, once someone is on sleeping pills, no matter how mild, it may be very difficult to get off them, because the body so rapidly gets used to them. Although he may sleep very well while taking the pills, without them he may suffer from an insomnia that is worse than it was before he went onto medication.

Very often, patients will seek the advice of a complementary therapist not at the onset of the insomnia but after they have been on sleeping pills for some time and have experienced difficulty in coming off them. Some acupuncturists maintain that the effects of sleeping pills (and other tranquilizers) on the system counteract the effects of acupuncture to some extent, so they will ask patients to discontinue their pills even before they start treatment. And because the drugs are still in the patient's body, it may take a little while before the treatment starts to work—although if he perseveres, the patient will find that acupuncture not only helps him sleep but also speeds the rate at which he excretes the drugs. However, other acupuncturists will treat a patient while he is still taking pills, allowing him to come off them in his own time once he begins to feel the effects of the treatment.

Let us take as our example here a middle-aged man who has found it increasingly difficult to sleep over the past few months. When he does manage to fall asleep, he dreams a great deal. He says that as a result of his sleeplessness he gets dizzy, has an intermittent ringing in his ears, and is becoming very irritable. He is also getting pains in his back, which he attributes to his tossing and turning at night. His face is pale but his lips are red; his eyes look dull and his tongue is red and thin. His pulse is rapid and disappears upon pressure.

From the fact that this condition is affecting the patient's mind (with sleeplessness, dreams, and irritability), we can determine that his heart—the seat of the mind—has been affected. The irritability, red lips, and rapid pulse are all indicative of heat. Still, his pale face and disappearing pulse speak of a deficiency. Dullness of the eyes suggests a deficiency of yin in the kidney. As we saw in the case of the elderly lady with hypertension, dizziness can be caused by hyperactivity of the liver's yang, secondary to inadequate nourishment of yin by the kidney. A thin red tongue is indicative of a deficiency of yin producing internal heat due to the relative excess of yang.

The meridian that has, so to speak, gotten out of control here is the Heart meridian. According to the servant-master relationship, the Heart meridian is the servant of the Kidney meridian, so a deficiency in the latter could produce symptoms of overactivity or heat in the former. Treatment should therefore stimulate the function of the kidney while sedating the activity of the heart.

Table 15 shows some of the points that might be used to achieve this.

TABLE 15. INSOMNIA TREATMENT

Point	Name	Meaning	Location	Function
H 7	Shenmen	Door of the Mind	Along the crease of the wrist, above the little finger	Strengthens the heart Chi to regulate the mind
UB 15	Xinshu	Heart shu point	To the side of the spine, a little above the level of the armpit	Has control over the heart and is used to treat mental disturbances of various types
UB 23	Shenshu	Kidney shu point	To the side of the spine, at about the level of the waist	Strengthens the kidney Chi
K 3	Taixi	Great Canyon	On the inside of the ankle, in the depression beside the Achilles tendon	Controls mental problems that have arisen as a result of a disharmony between the kidney and the heart

FACIAL PARALYSIS

In Western medicine this condition is known as Bell's palsy. The facial nerve on one or the other side of the face suddenly becomes inflamed and swollen. The reason for this is unknown, and the problem is limited to a single nerve. Eighty-five percent of patients with Bell's palsy recover completely, but recovery can be a long process; it may take nine months or more before the nerve is working normally again.

Let us suppose that a forty-five-year-old man has come to the acupuncture clinic showing the usual signs of this condition: an inability to shut the eye completely on the affected side (let us say, the left), watering of that eye, drooping of the left corner of his mouth, and a paralysis of the facial muscles on the left side so that he can no longer smile, frown, or whistle. Upon examination the left side of his face appears slightly swollen, as does the area around his left eye. His tongue has a white coating, and his pulse is superficial in character and slow. As with all patients suffering from this condition, he says that it came on rapidly, over the course of a day or two.

In Chinese medicine paralysis of any type is attributed to a complete blockage of the flow of Chi and of blood. The suddenness of this attack's onset suggests that it was due to an invasion by wind. This diagnosis is supported by the puffiness of the patient's face and eye. The white coating on his tongue and his slow pulse indicate that cold has also been a factor in producing the obstruction to Chi. The aim of treatment, therefore, is to disperse the wind and cold, and to stimulate the circulation of blood and of Chi. Moxa may be used to warm the points.

Table 16 shows a selection of the many points that may be used in the treatment of this condition.

TABLE 16. FACIAL PARALYSIS TREATMENT

Point	Name	Meaning	Location	Function
St 2	Sibai	Four Bright-nesses	On the cheekbone, on a line running vertically down the midpoint of the eye	Eliminates wind; is said to improve the eyesight in all four directions
St 4	Dicang	Storehouse of Earth	At the corner of the mouth, through which the fruit of the earth enters the body	A local point specific for the treatment of facial paralysis
SJ 17	Yifeng	Wind Screen	In the depression behind the base of the ear	An important point for treating problems of the face and head; expels wind
GB 1	Tongziliao	Orbit Bone	In the depression next to the outer angle of the eye	Eliminates wind
GB 2	Tinghui	Gathering of Hearing	Just in front of the ear, at the joint of the jaw	A local point specific for the treatment of facial paralysis
GB 12	Wangu	Mastoid Bone	In the depression behind the ear, behind and below the mastoid bone	A local point specific for the treatment of facial paralysis
GB 20	Fengchi	Wind Pool	At the back of the neck, in the depression below the base of the skull	Eliminates wind and cold

HEATSTROKE

This condition used to be called sunstroke, and northern Europeans living in the tropics would never go outdoors without a hat on, in order to avoid the supposedly evil effects of the sun on their heads. However, it is not sunshine itself but the heat that it produces that causes this condition, particularly when the atmosphere is humid so that the patient cannot cool down through the evaporation of sweat. Here, Western medicine is in agreement with Chinese medicine: Heatstroke is caused by an invasion of summer heat, which is a fierce, damp heat.

If we picture a patient with this condition, he is flushed, thirsty, and slightly confused; he has a headache. His mouth is dry and his pulse is superficial, bounding in character, and rapid. The signs all point to invasion by heat, and the patient's confusion suggests that his heart (the seat of the mind) has been affected. The treatment is to disperse the heat.

Some of the points that might be used are shown in table 17.

TABLE 17. HEATSTROKE TREATMENT

Point	Name	Meaning	Location	Function
LI 4	Hegu	Valley Junction	On the back of the hand, in the angle between the thumb and forefinger	Eliminates heat; tranquilizes the mind
St 36	Zusanli	Three Li on Lower Limbs	Three li below the knee	Strengthens Chi; counteracts the effect of summer heat
UB 40	Weizhong (alternative name: Xuexi)	Crooked Center (Blood Leak)	At the center of the crease behind the knee	If the point is pricked to make it bleed, this helps eliminate heat, stimulate the flow of blood, and restore consciousness
P 6	Neiguan	Medial Pass	A little way above the crease on the front of the wrist, along the midline of the forearm	Can be pricked to eliminate heat
P 7	Daling	Large Mound	In the middle of the crease on the front of the wrist	Has a similar function to P 6, and can be used with it to reinforce its effect
P 8	Laogong	Center of Work	In the center of the palm of the hand	Has a similar function to P 6, and can be used with it to reinforce its effect

GASTROENTERITIS

This is another condition most likely to affect people who are visiting hot countries. In fact, it is so common that there are now a number of medications available over the counter in drugstores that are specifically advertised as helpful in combating vacation stomach bugs. Let us say that the patient is a young man who is having a two-week vacation in Spain. After a couple of days he has developed abdominal pain and is passing hot, yellow, loose, and smelly stools that burn his anus as he passes them. He has a slight fever and is sweating. He has vomited a couple of times, and although he does not feel able to eat, he keeps on drinking water because he is thirsty most of the time. He has a sweet taste in his mouth that the water does not wash away. Upon examination his face is flushed and his lips are dry, despite the continual sips of water. His tongue is red with sticky a yellow coating, and his pulse is rapid with a slippery or gliding feel.

The passage of smelly, loose, yellow stools is indicative of an invasion of the spleen, stomach, and intestines by damp heat. The normal extraction of Chi from food by the stomach and spleen has been disrupted, and the circulation of Chi has become disordered; it is this that causes the vomiting. The fever and thirst, together with the patient's flushed face and red tongue, confirm the involvement of heat. A sweet taste in the mouth is associated with problems in the earth organs—the stomach and spleen—and their meridians, while dry lips are also indicative of heat in the spleen. A rapid pulse, of course, signifies heat, while its forceful, slippery quality implies an invasion of the digestive tract by damp, which is blocking the digestive process. Treatment aims to eliminate the damp heat and restore the stomach, spleen, and intestines to normal working order.

Table 18 shows some of the points that might be used to treat this patient.

TABLE 18. GASTROENTERITIS

Point	Name	Meaning	Location	Function
LI 4	Hegu	Valley Junction	On the back of the hand, in the angle between the thumb and forefinger	Eliminates heat
St 25	Tianshu	Axis of Heaven	On the abdomen, lying between the region above the navel (pertaining to heaven and yang) and that below it (pertaining to earth and yin)	Regulates the function of the stomach and intestines by eliminating damp and strengthening Chi
Sp 9	Yinlingquan	Yin Hill Spring	On the medial aspect of the leg, just below the knee	Eliminates damp; strengthens the spleen
UB 25	Dachang-shu	Large intestine shu point	Lateral to the spine, at about the level of the top of the hipbone	Stimulates the large intestine and its meridian
P 6	Neiguan	Medial Pass	A little way above the crease of the wrist, along the midline of the forearm	Eliminates heat; acts through its association with its fellow Fire meridian, the Sanjiao, whose middle section contains the stomach and spleen
Ren 12	Zhongwan	Middle of Stomach	Along the midline of the abdomen, a little way above the umbilicus	The mu, or alarm, point of the stomach, used to eliminate heat and damp from the stomach and spleen

BED-WETTING

All children who wet the bed grow out of the habit eventually, but some take longer than others. When the condition continues beyond the age of three or four, it can be a great nuisance, not only to the parents who have to change and wash the sheets but also to the child, who may become very anxious about his inability to stop. There are various Western treatments available, such as buzzers—electronic devices that are sensitive to damp. As soon as the child starts to wet the bed, the buzzer goes off and wakes him up. Some children find this very effective. Imipramine, a drug used as an antidepressant in adults, is another effective treatment, but naturally some parents do not wish their children to take drugs unless it is absolutely unavoidable. Of course, some children respond to neither of these treatments and require an alternative form of therapy to help them to stop wetting the bed. For them, acupuncture may prove very useful.

In Chinese medicine bed-wetting is seen as a lack of control over the urine due to a deficiency in the Water (Kidney and Urinary Bladder) meridians, and treatment is aimed at strengthening these. Table 19 shows some of the points that could be used for this treatment.

TABLE 19. BED-WETTING TREATMENT

Point	Name	Meaning	Location	Function
UB 23	Shenshu	Kidney shu point	To the side of the spine, at about the level of the waist	Strengthens the Chi of the kidney
UB 28	Pangguang-shu	Bladder shu point	To the side of the spine, in the sacral region (the lowest part of the spine)	Strengthens the Chi of the bladder
Ren 3	Zhongji	Exact Center	At the "center" of the body, along the midline of the abdomen, a short way above the pubic bone	A major point for treating disorders of the urinary tract
Ren 4	Guanyuan	Storage Place of Chi	On the midline of the abdomen, above Ren 3	Strengthens the kidney
Ren 6	Qihai	Sea of Chi	On the abdomen, on the midline, above Ren 4 and a little way below the umbilicus	Strengthens the kidney

IMPOTENCE

This is another condition in which the kidney is involved. In Chinese medicine the kidney is thought to be responsible for governing the reproductive system, so any abnormalities in a patient's sexual function are said to stem from problems relating to the kidney. Since impotence may be seen as a form of deficiency, with aspects of internalization and lack of movement, the element that would be deficient is yang, resulting in a relative excess of yin. The deficiency may involve not only the Kidney meridian but also the Ren meridian (or Vessel of Conception)—the midline channel running down the front of the body. The Ren meridian is associated with the sexual organs because of its pathway. Treatment of impotence consists primarily of stimulation of the yang of the kidney in order to restore balance.

Possible points for the treatment of impotence are shown in table 20.

TABLE 20. IMPOTENCE TREATMENT

Point	Name	Meaning	Location	Function
UB 23	Shenshu	Kidney shu point	To the side of the spine, at about the level of the waist	A major point for treating disorders of the urogenital system; used for its direct effect on the kidney
Du 4	Mingmen	Gate of Life	Along the midline of the back, at the level of the kidney	An important point for reinforcing the yang of the kidney
Du 20	Baihui	Many Meetings	At the crossing point of the Urinary Bladder, Liver, and Du meridians, on the crown of the head	Regulates and activates yang Chi
Ren 3	Zhongji	Exact Center	At the "center" of the body, along the midline of the abdomen, a short way above the pubic bone	A major point for treating disorders of the urogenital system; used for its direct effect on the kidney
Ren 4	Guanyuan	Storage Place of Chi	On the midline of the abdomen, above Ren 3	Moxibustion of this point strengthens the yang of the kidney

FEBRILE CONVULSIONS

Certain children are prone to have fits if they develop infections that cause their temperatures to rise rapidly. Fortunately, it is a susceptibility that most grow out of after the age of about two, and usually the fits are short lived and therefore not life threatening. However, they are extremely worrying for the parents, who have to be constantly aware of the problem. In order to try to avoid further episodes of convulsions they have to start tepid-sponging the child and giving him acetaminophen as soon as he shows any signs of developing a fever.

Let us imagine an eighteen-month-old girl who, having caught a cold a few days previously, has suddenly developed a high fever and had a fit, during which she has gone blue for a few seconds. Upon examination following the fit she is flushed and has a rapid pulse that feels wiry. A sudden onset of disease always suggests the involvement of wind, while the fever and rapid pulse indicate the presence of heat. Cyanosis (going blue) suggests that the liver is involved, since this is the organ responsible for the normal circulation of Chi. The treatment is to eliminate both heat and wind, which can be effected by using some of the points shown in table 21.

Naturally, when treating a small child, the number of needles is kept to a minimum. The points described here would never be used all at the same time.

TABLE 21. FEBRILE CONVULSION TREATMENT

Point	Name	Meaning	Location	Function
LI 1	Shangyan	Yang Shang (shang is the sound associated with metal and its meridians)	On the thumb side of the index finger, near the corner of the nail	Expels wind
LI 4	Hegu	Valley Junction	On the back of the hand, in the angle between the thumb and forefinger	Removes heat; clears obstructions to the flow of Chi; specifically relieves convulsions
LI 11	Quchi	Crooked Pool	In a depression at the lateral side of the elbow crease	Expels wind; is an important point for the treatment of fever
SI 3	Houxi	Back Brook	In a depression on the little-finger side of the hand, just above the line of the knuckles	Removes heat and relieves spasm by tranquilizing the mind
K 1	Yongquan	Bubbling Spring	In the depression on the sole of the foot, from where the Chi of the meridian bubbles upward	An important point for treating infantile convulsions
P 8	Laogong	Center of Work	In the center of the palm of the hand	Removes heat and relieves spasm by tranquilizing the mind
GB 34	Yangling-quan	Yang Mound Spring	In a depression below the bony prominence on the outer aspect of the knee	Promotes the flow of Chi; is an important point for treating infantile convulsions
Liv 2	Xingjian	Walking Between	Between the first and second toes	Dispels heat from the liver to prevent wind from being generated internally
Liv 3	Taichong	Great Pass	On the upper aspect of the foot, along a line that runs between the first and second toes	Dispels heat from the liver to prevent wind from being generated internally; often used with LI 4

NOSEBLEEDS

Some people are troubled by recurring nosebleeds. Usually the bleeding occurs from an area at the back of the nose, known as Little's area, which is particularly well supplied with tiny blood vessels. These vessels may become fragile and bleed at the slightest provocation. If the nosebleeds become very frequent or severe, Western medicine offers cauterization of Little's area. This is a fairly minor procedure, and it usually stops further bleeding. Medication is also available that, if taken at the time of a nosebleed, will help shut down these tiny blood vessels.

However, let us look at a patient who has not tried Western treatment and has arrived at the acupuncture clinic just after having had a nosebleed. Upon examination he looks slightly flushed, and his pulse is rapid. Hemorrhage is often due to invasion by heat. The nose is the sense organ that is associated with the lung, so we can deduce from the patient's symptoms that there is an excess of heat in the Lung meridian, which is corroborated by the patient's pulse and his flushed appearance. Treatment consists in eradicating the heat.

Table 22 shows some of the points that might be used.

The combination of UB 60 and K 3 can be used to stop a current nosebleed due to heat arising as a result of a relative excess of yang caused by a deficiency kidney yin. This can be used as a first-aid measure, since pressure on the two points works just as well. An acupuncturist may instruct his patient on the exact location of these points for emergency use.

TABLE 22. NOSEBLEED TREATMENT

Point	Name	Meaning	Location	Function
Lu 11	Shaoshang	Minor Shang (shang is the sound associated with metal and its meridians)	Near the corner of the thumbnail	Clears heat from the lung
LI 4	Hegu	Valley Junction	On the back of the hand, in the angle between the thumb and forefinger	An important point for treating diseases of the lung (the large intestine and lung are both metal, so they have close affinity); in this case it would be used to expel heat from the lung
UB 60	Kunlun	A mountain range in Tibet	On the lateral aspect of the ankle, between the Achilles tendon and the anklebone	Clears heat from the lung
K 3	Taixi	Great Canyon	On the medial aspect of the ankle, in the depression beside the Achilles tendon	Clears heat from the lung

SOME CASE HISTORIES

I wish to thank Dr. Peter Helps of Brighton, England; Mr. Roger Murray of Lewes, England; and their patients for allowing me to quote some of the following case histories.

Mrs. G. M.

This middle-aged woman first saw an acupuncturist during the month of February. The previous September she had stretched her right arm back to pick something up and felt a tearing pain in her shoulder. It had subsided after a few minutes and she thought no more of it until it started up again some days later, this time lasting for three weeks. After this she was free of pain until November, when it returned and gradually became worse, spreading to affect her upper arm as well. She was unable to lie on her right side at night; if she stretched her arm above her head while she was asleep, the pain would wake her up, sweating and gasping for breath.

Mrs. G. M. went to see her doctor and was told that what she had was a frozen shoulder. The doctor added that there was little treatment he could offer. Steroid injections or manipulation under anesthetic were sometimes used, but these had been known to make matters worse in some cases. If left alone, the condition should resolve in about two years, so his advice was to take painkillers and wait.

Mrs. G. M. worked as a librarian in the local university library, so she had to be able to lift heavy books and sometimes put them onto high shelves. Since she could no longer raise her arm higher than the horizontal, she could not do her job. She could not have two years' sick leave; either she had to find a cure or lose her job. One of her friends recommended an acupuncturist, to whom she went with some trepidation.

Upon examination Mrs. G. M. was found to have a wiry pulse, indicating a stagnation of blood and Chi. Because of the location of the pain, a diagnosis was made of stagnation in the Large Intestine, Small Intestine, and Sanjiao meridians. Mrs. G. M.'s tongue had cracks in the center and at the sides, suggesting a yin deficiency. In all, Mrs. G. M. had eight sessions of treatment, during which the points detailed in table 23 were used.

TABLE 23. MRS. G. M.'S TREATMENT

Point	Name	Meaning	Location	Function
Lu 2	Yunmen	Cloud Door	In the hollow below the outer end of the collarbone	Used for its local effect on the shoulder
Lu 7	Lieque	Broken Clouds	Above the bony prominence on the thumb side of the wrist	Strengthens the Chi of the lung
LI 4	Hegu	Valley Junction	On the back of the hand, in the angle between the thumb and forefinger	Relieves stagnation of Chi
LI 15	Jianyu	Corner of Shoulder	Just below the point of the shoulder	Specific for pain in the shoulder joint
LI 16	Jugu	Huge Bone (the ancient Chinese name for the collarbone)	On the ridge of the shoulder	Used for its local effect on the shoulder
Sp 6	Sanyinjiao	Three Yin Meridians Crossing	On the medial aspect of the leg, a short way above the ankle, at the intersection point of the Spleen, Liver, and Kidney meridians	Stimulates yin
SI 10	Naoshu	Point at Muscle Prominence	At the back of the shoulder joint	Specific for pain in the shoulder joint
K 6	Zhaohai	Shining Sea	On the inner aspect of the ankle	Opens the yin Ren meridian to help counteract yin deficiency
SJ 5	Waiguan	Lateral Pass	A short distance above SJ 4 on the lateral side of the humerus bone	Relieves stagnation of Chi
SJ 14	Jianliao	Shoulder Opening	In a hollow below the bone at the back of the shoulder	Specific for pain in the shoulder joint
GB 21	Jianjing	Well of the Shoulder	Where the base of the neck joins the shoulder	Dispels wind
GB 34	Yanglingquan	Yang Mound Spring	In a depression below the bony prominence on the lateral aspect of the knee	Dispels wind; clears damp heat; stimulates liver yin*

*Liver yin nourishes the joints so, by improving this, you can improve mobility.

At the first session the acupuncturist used three local points to treat the pain—SJ 14, LI 15, and SI 10; two points to move the stagnation—LI 4 and SJ 5; and Sp 6 to treat the yin deficiency. The patient was asked to return at weekly intervals.

At her next appointment Mrs. G. M. reported that the pain was not quite so bad, and she was sleeping a little better. Upon examination her pulse was found to be less wiry. The acupuncturist used the same points as before, along with an additional local point, LI 16. The problem seemed to be due to an external rather than an internal disharmony, and it was at this that the main treatment was aimed.

The following week the patient reported that, although the pain was less severe, she had had a menstrual period that lasted for twelve days. Her pulse was found to be deficient. Because Chi is extracted and refined from the air in the chest, Lung meridian points can be used to nourish the whole body. In states of Lung meridian deficiency, the shoulder is especially vulnerable to problems. Because there was now a suggestion of an internal, Lung, deficiency, some points were used to nourish the interior, although the main treatment was still external. The local points treated were Lu 2, SI 10, and SJ 14. Needles were also put in the distal points Lu 7 and K 6.

By the next appointment Mrs. G. M. was feeling much better and was finding it easier to move her arm. She had also noticed that the athlete's foot that she had had for many years was beginning to clear up. The treatment from the previous week was repeated, with the addition of LI 16.

On her fifth visit the patient was found to have a "soggy" pulse and a thin white coating on her tongue, both indicating the presence of damp heat. The previous treatment was repeated, together with a needle in GB 34.

By April Mrs. G. M. was reporting good days and bad days. The pain that had originally been sharp (indicating a stagnation of blood) had given way to a dull ache (indicating stagnation of Chi). This was a definite improvement, because stagnation of blood is seen as being a symptom of a deeper disharmony than is stagnation of Chi. The pain was no longer in one place but tended to move around, suggesting invasion by wind—which classically affects the two Wood meridians, Liver and Gall Bladder. To remedy this, a local point, GB 21, and a distal point, GB 34 were used in addition to the regular treatment.

By May, after eight sessions with the acupuncturist, Mrs. G. M. was free of pain, had regained almost all the movement in her arm, and was able to return to work.

Mrs. C. B.

Mrs. C. B. was a menopausal woman who went to see an acupuncturist for the first time during a heat wave in August. She had been having hot flashes for some time, which had not troubled her too much, but since the heat wave had begun she had been finding them intolerable.

At menopause there is said to be a decline in Jing, or essence. Jing is one of the three treasures of Chinese medicine, the others being Shen (spirit) and Chi. Jing is said to program the whole cycle of growth, maturation, and decline. When it begins to decrease around menopause, it sets up an imbalance between yin and yang. Hot flashes (particularly at night, when yin should be at its strongest) are a manifestation of excessive yang, as is the restlessness that they usually cause.

Upon examination Mrs. C. B.'s tongue showed cracks, suggesting a yin deficiency, and her pulse was deficient at the deep levels, indicating a deficiency in the interior, yin organs. Mrs. C. B. had four sessions of treatment during which the points detailed in table 24 were used.

TABLE 24. MRS. C. B.'S TREATMENT

Point	Name	Meaning	Location	Function
Lu 7	Lieque	Broken Clouds	Above the bony prominence on the thumb side of the wrist	Strengthens Chi; nourishes yin
St 36	Zusanli	Three Li on Lower Limbs	Three li below the knee	Strengthens Chi; nourishes yin
Sp 6	Sanyinjiao	Three Yin Meridians Crossing	On the lateral aspect of the leg, a short way above the ankle, at the intersection point of the Spleen, Liver, and Kidney meridians	Nourishes yin
K 6	Zhaohai	Shining Sea	On the inner aspect of the ankle	Opens the yin Ren meridian to help counteract yin deficiency by making the yin in the Ren available to the rest of the body

After two sessions Mrs. C. B. was much better. Two further sessions at six-month intervals were all she needed to see her through menopause.

Mr. B. V.

This twenty-four-year-old man woke up one morning to find that he was unable to move his right wrist. He could use his arm perfectly normally, but his right hand hung limply and could not be raised. This condition, known as wrist drop, is usually due to injury or prolonged pressure affecting the nerve supply to the muscles of the forearm and hand. However, in Mr. B. V.'s case, no such history was forthcoming.

He was seen by the neurology specialist at the local hospital, and a diagnosis of localized nerve damage was made. The only explanation seemed to be that Mr. B. V. must have lain in such a position while asleep that the nerve was stretched or damaged. Whatever the cause, though, the neurologist told him that there was no specific treatment; he would just have to wait for the nerve to recover, something that could take between six months and two years. Meanwhile he was to have physiotherapy, which would prevent the affected muscles from contracting.

TABLE 25. MR. B. V.'S TREATMENT

Point	Name	Meaning	Location	Function
Lu 7	Liequeq	Broken Clouds	Above the bony prominence on the thumb side of the wrist	Expels wind; a specific point for treating weakness or paralysis in the wrist
LI 4	Hegu	Valley Junction	On the back of the hand, in the angle between the thumb and forefinger	Expels wind
SI 4	Wangu	Wristbone	On the side of the wrist, above the little finger	A specific point for treating weakness or paralysis in the wrist
SJ 4	Yangchi	Pool of Yang	On the back of the wrist	Stimulates the flow of Chi; removes obstructions; also used for its local effects on the hand and wrist
SJ 5	Waiguan	Lateral Pass	A short distance above SJ 4 on the lateral side of the humerus bone	Relieves stagnation of Chi

It was the physiotherapist who suggested that acupuncture might help and, accordingly, Mr. B. V. went for treatment. A sudden paralysis of this nature suggests an obstruction to the flow of Chi due to invasion by wind. Only local points were used, as detailed in table 25.

The patient was treated every other day for two weeks, after which he had recovered a considerable amount of movement in his wrist. He continued to have treatment twice a week and within six weeks was back to normal.

Mr. J. A.

Mr. J. A. was a man of forty-three who, twenty years earlier, having taken a degree in geology at an English university, was offered a job with a large firm in Australia. He leaped at the chance of seeing the world and undertook his new job with great enthusiasm. For a time everything went very well. He was competent and well liked by the men with whom he worked. He met an Australian woman, and they planned to get married. However, one day there was a very serious accident at his worksite: two men were badly mutilated.

It fell to Mr. J. A. to write out the reports of these accidents, and while he was doing so his right arm suddenly stopped functioning. He could grip the pen with his hand but was quite unable to move his arm. He saw the company doctor, who could not explain what had happened except to suggest that it might be some localized form of polio. After several weeks there was no sign of recovery, and eventually Mr. J. A. lost his job on the grounds of chronic incapacity. He was thoroughly depressed by this and even more so by the fact that no one could tell him what had caused the problem or whether it was ever likely to get better. He was unable to face looking for another job in a country that was not his home so, breaking his engagement, he left for England.

Back home he found it hard to get a job and had to take whatever he could get. But he remained unsettled. His arm was not improving, and the muscles were beginning to atrophy. After a succession of jobs that offered him no mental challenge, he decided to start his own business. It was around this time, too, that he met an English woman and married her.

Unfortunately, he was dogged by bad luck. Eventually his business capsized, and he was left with serious financial problems. He struggled on but was having difficulties at home as well. He and his wife were not getting along; they finally divorced. He found a job but, as before, it was no challenge to him. This, together with his divorce and financial problems, produced a severe depression, and he became suicidal.

At the height of these problems and upon the recommendation of a friend, he decided to have some acupuncture treatment. The acupuncturist who treated him was a practitioner of the Five Elements school. He diagnosed Mr. J. A. as having an imbalance in his Earth meridians. This was based on the fact that his face appeared to have yellow lines, his voice was singing in character, and he craved sympathy. In addition, the acupuncturist was impressed by the patient's great interest in geology and things of the earth. The Earth meridians are those of the Spleen and the Stomach; upon taking Mr. J. A.'s pulses the two corresponding to these meridians were found to be bounding.

The treatment comprised sedation of the meridians that were in excess, together with transfer of Chi from them to deficient meridians by the use of specific transfer points. In addition, the source points of the Stomach and Spleen meridians were used, because these are the direct links to the stomach and spleen themselves. The element points—that is, the Earth points—on both meridians were also used.

After two months of treatment, although there was as yet no noticeable difference in his arm, the patient's whole attitude toward life started to change. The depression left him, and he started to think in a far more positive manner than before. He began to talk about returning to Australia and seeing if he could find his fiancée of twenty years before. After four months he started to regain some movement in his arm and was referred by his general practitioner to the local hospital for physiotherapy.

After nine months of treatment Mr. J. A. returned to Australia. Two months later his acupuncturist received a letter saying that he had met up again with his first fiancée. She had married a year after he had left Australia, but her marriage, too, had failed. They were intending to get married shortly and make up for lost time. His arm, he said, was continuing to improve, and he was hoping to find an acupuncturist in Adelaide where they were settling so that he could continue treatment.

Mr. D. K.

This forty-five-year-old man telephoned the acupuncturist one Friday afternoon asking for an emergency appointment. He had a severe toothache and needed some treatment to control the pain until he could see his dentist on the following Monday morning.

His history was an interesting one. He had been a high-powered executive in a large company for a number of years, and the pressures under which he worked were enormous. His sphere of responsibility gradually grew until, to relieve the stress, he started to drink. His alcohol intake increased until he was drinking a bottle of whiskey or more a day. By this time it was the alcohol that was making it impossible for him to cope with his job, and he was replaced.

After this trauma he found another job and managed to stop drinking with the aid of Alcoholics Anonymous, but his body began to react to all the various stresses that he had been under and he developed allergies. At first he reacted only to common allergens such as pollen and cat fur. Then he began to find that certain foods would make him vomit. Finally substances such as diesel fumes began to affect him so that he was unable to walk along a busy road without feeling sick and faint.

He went to see a specialist at the local hospital and was started on a course of desensitizing injections. He was warned that the course of treatment could be a long one, since he seemed to be allergic to so many substances. When he developed a toothache, he knew that he would be unable to visit the dentist immediately—he would be affected by the anesthetic gases present in the air of the dentist's office that had accumulated during the week. The only answer was to get an appointment for first thing Monday morning, when the office would be relatively gas-free. Meanwhile, he wanted some acupuncture to control the pain.

Now, acupuncture can be used for emergency treatment, but the best results are achieved when a course of treatment is given. The reason for this is that acupuncture involves manipulating energies; although temporary relief can be obtained from one treatment, problems may occur at a later date if the energies are not completely returned to normal. So when Mr. D. K. called for an emergency acupuncture appointment, he was told that he could only be seen if he agreed to come for a follow-up course of treatment.

This was acceptable to Mr. D. K., and his toothache was treated by the insertion of two needles. The pain was relieved for thirty-six hours and, on Monday, he saw his dentist. When he returned to the acupuncturist, a diagnosis was made according to the Law of the Five Elements. Mr. D. K. showed grief and anguish when he talked about his problems and his voice had a weeping quality, indicating that the element that was out of balance was metal. However, his face had a bluish look to it and his bodily smell seemed putrid, suggesting that there were problems with the water element as well. The acupuncturist diagnosed a deficiency in both elements. Water is the child of metal, and deficiency in the mother can produce an undernourished child—the so-called screaming child syndrome.

The treatment consisted of stimulating the deficient metal using primarily the element points (that is, the Metal points on the Large Intestine and Lung meridians, which are the Metal meridians) and also the source points on the Metal meridians.

By his fourth treatment there had been a noticeable improvement, and Mr. D. K. spoke to the consultant at the hospital about the necessity of continuing with his allergy injections. As a result these were gradually reduced. After four months of acupuncture treatment he had stopped the injections altogether, and all trace of his allergies had disappeared.

Mr. P. S.

Mr. P. S. was a thirty-two-year-old policeman who had joined the force some eight years earlier, after coming out of the army. Although he enjoyed his job, he found it stressful, and for the past three years he had been taking tranquilizers regularly.

He had coped with a number of fairly traumatic incidents in his earlier life, including a very severe accident at the age of twenty-one, when he was knocked off his motorcycle. He had been in intensive care for three months following this but ultimately made a full recovery and was able to return to his army duties. When he was twenty-five he had been posted to Northern Ireland for two years and, during his time there, had seen a friend badly injured. He himself had narrowly escaped being killed as well.

All this stress had taken its toll, and Mr. P. S. had become a chain smoker. And, although his job with the police force was far less stressful than his previous work, he had much less resistance than before. He had recurrent attacks of severe pain in his chest and back, along with shivering. On two occasions he had been rushed to hospital with a presumed heart attack. The tranquilizers did not seem to reduce his symptoms, but he was scared of going without them, in case things got even worse. He described himself as being full of fear.

Mr. P. S. had reached the stage where he could see that, sooner or later, he would not be able to carry on with his job. He decided to look for help and, on the advice of a colleague, made an appointment for some acupuncture, with the idea of trying to get rid of his chest pain.

He was diagnosed, in accordance with the Law of the Five Elements, as having problems relating to metal. This was based on the weeping quality of his voice, the anguish and grief with which he told his story, the white appearance of his face, and his putrid body smell. However, the acupuncturist also determined that he was suffering from a complete obstruction to the circulation of Chi. He therefore started treatment with a combination of needles known as the Treatment of the Seven Dragons. This is used specifically in cases of a severe disruption of energy flow affecting the whole body, and it is interesting to note that the position of several of the needles used in this correspond to the positions of the major chakras, or psychic energy centers of the body. (Energy medicine, like acupuncture, is based on the manipulation of energy flow.) After the treatment Mr. P. S. started to tremble. This became quite severe and continued for about forty-five minutes after the needles had been removed.

Follow-up treatments consisted of strengthening the heart and the Heart meridian: The heart is associated with fire, and metal is the servant of fire, so weakness of fire can result in it losing control of metal. The Metal source points and element points were also used.

The results were remarkable. After only a few treatments Mr. P. S. was able to stop taking his tranquilizers. After several months he had lost all his anxiety and was enjoying life to the full.

8

Acupuncture and Modern Science

We live today in a scientific and materialistic world in which everything has to be proved before it can be believed. Many people have difficulty accepting anything that cannot readily be explained except in its own terms. And charlatans and forgers over the years have helped to make skeptics of us all. Complementary medicine has suffered greatly in this respect. To those of us who have been brought up in the West, in an environment of hospitals and health maintenance organizations, doctors and dentists, the complementary therapies—particularly some of the more "way out" ones—seem to be in much the same category as fortune-telling and UFOs.

One of the main stumbling blocks to a wider acceptance of complementary therapies is the fact that they use a completely different vocabulary from Western medicine and science. The terms in which acupuncture is explained and the concepts of Chi and of the meridians are not easily assimilated into Western thinking. To suggest to a Western-trained scientist that acupuncture works by the manipulation of (to him) unproven body energies is as convincing as saying that a conjuring trick works because the magician says, "Abracadabra." In short, acupuncture is unscientific. Although more and more Western physicians are becoming aware that acupuncture works, many of them are unable to accept the terms in which it is explained. And so these physicians, wishing to use acupuncture

165

but not understanding it, have felt obliged to "explain" its workings in their own terminology.

There is, of course, nothing intrinsically wrong in this. If you wish a Frenchman who speaks only his mother tongue to appreciate a book that has been written in English, you must translate it into French. This is perfectly acceptable. It starts to become a problem, however, when the Frenchman declares that until the works of Shakespeare, Jane Austen, and Chaucer have been translated into French, they are of no value. It is quite understandable that Western physicians should wish to know how acupuncture works in their own terms—that is, related to the nervous system and physiology as they know it. However, there are those who maintain that until such a time as it has been proven to them empirically that the insertion of needles into acupuncture points results in measurable changes in the patient's physiology, they will regard acupuncture as suspect.

Anyone who has taken the time to look at acupuncture will tell you there is no doubt that it works. And patients who have been treated with acupuncture and consequently recovered from illnesses for which Western practitioners had nothing to offer will tell you that they don't care how it works. Acupuncture has shown over a period of two thousand years and more that it works. Scientific investigation of its workings should not be deemed essential in order to corroborate this fact.

Many of the investigations that have been carried out into acupuncture in the West have been based on the premise that it is the anatomically demonstrable nervous system, rather than any hypothetical system of meridians, that is responsible for the results achieved by the therapy. It must be said, however, that physicians still do not fully understand the workings of the nervous system, which is the most complex system of the body. So scientifc experiments designed to demonstrate pseudo-acupuncture effects are doing so only in the light of an incompletely understood system.

Of course, in none of these experiments is any attention paid to the concept of the life force. This doesn't come into physiology at all. While we are building bigger and better machines and computers that become more and more like humans, able to take over our work and perhaps to do it even better than we do, we are also reducing humanity itself to the level of a machine. There comes a point, however, at which both tendencies—the building up of the machines and the reduction of humanity—reach an impasse from which they cannot escape, simply because there will always be the difference that a live man or woman is permeated by a life force; when that force goes, the body dies. A machine has no such force and therefore can be repaired almost ad infinitum, providing that replacement parts are available. You can carry on replacing parts of a machine until there is nothing of the original left—yet, fundamentally, it is the same machine. You cannot do that with a living being.

Such a concept does seem to take us into the realms of theology, since the life force can be compared with what theologians would call spirit. Much science fiction has been written about the creation of living beings by man. But although animals have been successfully cloned, and although it is possible to manufacture protein and the other components of humans in a test tube, no one has found out how to create a living thing from first principles. The life force remains elusive.

The idea of the merging of disciplines—of bridging the gap between chemistry and biology, between botany and zoology, even between theology and science—takes us back to the idea of holism, which is the basis of so many complementary therapies. A colleague of mine once observed that many Western practitioners are valiantly trying to adopt the concept of holism but, to them, it means taking account not only of the body but also of the mind and spirit, whereas, of course, true holism entails just looking at the *patient*. Body, mind, and spirit form a whole, and just because the first of these can be more fully explained than the other two—and the last can be explained not at all—does not mean they can be divided from each other.

Having said all that, it can do no harm to ask how acupuncture is related to physiology as understood by Western physicians. Many of the experiments that demonstrate the workings of the nervous system are performed on animals (a highly controversial issue in itself). These have shown us that stimulation of certain points on the skin can produce effects at a distance from these points that seem to be dependent on the normal functioning of the nervous system. Because animal experimentation permits the destruction of various parts of the animal's nervous system, we also have been able to find out which part of the system carries the signal. What is interesting is that in the nervous-system theory of acupuncture, depending on which part of the body is stimulated, the nervous impulses that seem to be responsible for producing the effect appear to be carried in different ways. It is therefore difficult to propound an overall theory explaining in Western terms how acupuncture works.

For example, experiments have been performed in which stimulation of the skin on the back of rats produced changes in their intestines. The results were found to be the same whether a rat's nervous system was intact or its spinal cord had been divided, cutting off the body from the brain. From this it was deduced that the brain was not involved, and that all the nervous impulses controlling the effects of stimulation were carried by the spinal cord. However, a similar experiment performed on fish, where stimulation of the lower part of the bowel produced changes in the skin, was found to be effective even if the spinal cord had been destroyed. In this case a different mechanism seemed to be involved, the effects apparently being produced by the sympathetic nervous system.

In his book *Acupuncture: The Ancient Chinese Art of Healing,* Felix Mann puts forward the theory that the responses obtained in various organs of the body when points on the skin are stimulated tie in with the way in which the body develops as an embryo. Each section of the body, together with its nerve supply, develops from a different section of the embryo. Physicians call these sections dermatomes. Very often both an organ and the acupuncture points that affect it lie in the same dermatome. However, Mann points out that the "acupuncture points of the legs and head do not fit in with what is known of dermatomes." This means that another theory has to be found to explain how acupuncture works in these parts of the body.

While the medical profession struggles to understand how acupuncture works, acupuncture as a method of pain relief has become quite respectable thanks to the discovery of endorphins.

Endorphins are substances produced by the body that have the effect of controlling pain. Secretion of large amounts of endorphins occurs automatically in response to severe pain—for instance, during childbirth and after serious injury. It would appear that the level of endorphins circulating in the bloodstream under normal conditions varies from person to person. This may explain why different people have different pain thresholds, some being able to tolerate pain far more readily than others.

Stimulation of acupuncture points that produce anesthetic effects has been shown to release endorphins into the body. What has not been explained—at least not in Western terms—is why stimulation of these particular points and no others produces these effects.

A colleague of mine once said that the discovery of endorphins was the best thing that had ever happened to acupuncture, because it enabled the medical profession to accept the technique's validity. "Western thought," she said, "has got this wonderful ability to say that if you can't explain it, it doesn't exist." Very true, yet, this attitude is rather odd when you consider that, as far as I am aware, no one has yet explained fully the way in which aspirin works, nor some of the antidepressants, nor many of the drugs that are handed out day after day in general practitioners' offices. On the whole, the basic biochemical action of such drugs is understood—how each reacts in the body and what the effects of those reactions are. But in many cases the ways in which those chemical reactions produce the final effects felt by the patient are poorly understood. Nevertheless, the medical profession is satisfied that each drug produces the same effect time and time again, and therefore it is used for that purpose. When it comes to acupuncture, however, the fact that certain treatments can produce certain results time and time again is disregarded because "we don't know how it works."

Of course, this attitude is not representative of the entire medical profession. Many of its members are now becoming very interested in complementary therapies and are coming around to the view that "if it works and is safe, then it should be used, even if we don't fully understand how it works." It is indeed very difficult for a Western practitioner, brought up in the realms of things that he can see and measure—nerves producing electrical impulses, red blood cells carrying measurable amounts of oxygen, kidney cells secreting waste products into the urine—to accept things that cannot be seen or measured but just have to be taken on trust.

In one way it is easier to accept acupuncture than it is to accept some of the other complementary therapies. The acupuncture meridians can be seen as the ancient Chinese description of the nervous system, and the effects of acupuncture may, to an extent, be explained as functions of the nervous system. The theories on which energy medicines, radionics, and homeopathy are founded are much harder for a Western physician to understand. However, practitioners of these systems would find it relatively easy to accept the philosophy of acupuncture. In energy therapies and radionics, for example, energy is said to flow through a system of nadis—a fine network of channels that pervades and surrounds the entire body. Thus it is easy for a healer to understand the system of meridians as an aspect of the nadis and for the acupuncturist to understand the nadis as an extension of the meridians. In the end it may well be acupuncture that brings together the practitioners of Eastern and Western therapies by having a component that both sides can understand or relate to.

Attitudes are changing, and more and more Western practitioners are referring patients to acupuncturists and are even using acupuncture themselves (I shall say more about this in the next chapter). It is an important step forward. For, as a colleague once said, "If we all stood around waiting for things to be fully explained before we used them, we'd be watching television by candlelight!"

9

Finding Out about Treatment

The growing popularity of acupuncture in the West has meant that, for a number of years, it has been possible for aspiring practitioners to complete their training in their own country, although there are still some who opt to do at least part of their work in China. In North America a large number of colleges offer acupuncture training, including the American College of Acupuncture and Oriental Medicine in Texas (which offers a master of science degree in Oriental medicine), South Baylo University in California (which runs a four-year course in acupuncture and Oriental medicine, leading to a master of science degree), the Northwest Institute of Acupuncture and Oriental Medicine in Seattle (whose three-year course leads to a M.Ac. degree), the National College of Oriental Medicine in Florida (which runs a three-year degree course), and the International College of Traditional Chinese Medicine of Vancouver (which runs a four-year diploma course in traditional Chinese medicine as well as three-year diploma courses in Chinese acupuncture and Chinese herbology). The recognized accrediting agency for the approval of programs to train practitioners in acupuncture and Oriental medicine in the United States is the Accreditation Commission for Acupuncture and Oriental Medicine (ACAOM).

In Britain the British Acupuncture Council regulates the practice of acupuncture, although it does not have all the powers over the training and conduct of practitioners that the General Medical Council has over that of U.K. doctors. The various colleges teach in different ways and award their own qualifications. And there are numerous short courses available, especially for doctors, which offer no qualifications. Two of the main colleges in the United Kingdom are the College of Traditional Chinese Acupuncture in Leamington Spa, Warwickshire, which teaches the Five Elements system, and the International College of Oriental Medicine in East Grinstead, Sussex, which teaches the Eight Principles system. According to the length of time that they have studied acupuncture, graduates of the College of Traditional Chinese Acupuncture may put the letters Lic. Ac., B.Ac., M.Ac., or D.Ac. after their names. Graduates of the International College of Oriental Medicine may become B.Ac., M.Ac., or D.Ac. Among the other colleges are the South West College of Oriental Medicine in Bristol (which is affiliated with the Shanghai University of Traditional Chinese Medicine), the London School of Acupuncture and Traditional Chinese Medicine (which is part of the University of Westminster), and the College of Integrated Chinese Medicine in Reading. Ireland has the Irish College of Traditional Chinese Medicine in Dublin.

As is clear from this, acupuncture practitioners have a wide variety of training backgrounds. So to whom should you go for treatment? It might, on the whole, be easier to say to whom you should *not* go. As a rule of thumb for any of the complementary therapies, avoid practitioners who advertise. This is because the majority of governing bodies in the world of complementary therapies forbid practitioners registered with them to advertise. Thus if a practitioner advertises, it is often an indication that he is not fully trained and registered. This does not apply to a listing in the yellow pages, nor to a single announcement in a newspaper that a practitioner is now available to see patients. However, it does apply to newspaper advertisements, leaflets, or posters along the lines of DO YOU HAVE BACKACHE? MIGRAINE? ARTHRITIS? ACUPUNCTURE THERAPY WILL HELP.

One very good way of finding a practitioner is to ask around among your friends, because a personal recommendation is well worth having. Of course, as I have mentioned, some Western doctors now practice acupuncture in addition to Western medicine. A few will have completed the full three- or four-year training, but prospective patients should be aware that others have only taken short courses and use the treatment symptomatically—in other words, they are not concerned with the holistic application of balancing the patient's energies but only with alleviating his symptoms (usually pain). This may be perfectly acceptable if all you want is pain relief. In fact, many of the doctors who practice acupuncture are anesthetists and rheumatologists, who use it in their pain clinics. Doctors, too, are just as good at putting in ear studs to help smokers and dieters as anybody else.

However, if your problem is more complicated or if you feel that you need the holistic approach, make sure your acupuncturist uses either the system of the Five Elements or the system of the Eight Principles. If you call an acupuncturist with a view to making an appointment, it is quite appropriate to ask him which system he uses. Tell him your problem, briefly, and ask whether he thinks he can help. Sometimes it is advantageous to go to a therapist who is working in a natural therapies center since, if the acupuncturist does not think that he can help you, he may be able to refer you to a colleague whose therapy may suit you better, such as an herbalist, a homeopath, or an osteopath. Sometimes an acupuncturist may also practice other therapies, which can be beneficial. Occasionally two therapies together may work better than one alone. In my experience the effects of acupuncture can be increased when used together with manipulation or energy therapies.

Of course, like all therapies, acupuncture does not work for everybody. If you go to a reputable practitioner, however, you can be sure that he will not keep bringing you back if you are unlikely to respond. Depending on how long you have been ill, it may take a while before you begin to notice any great improvement, so it is important to be patient and not to give up on your treatments. Your acupuncturist ought to be able to tell you at which stage you should start thinking about trying another therapy if nothing seems to be happening. Some practitioners ask patients to commit themselves to a certain number of sessions in order to give the therapy a good chance of working. Usually, if you are going to get results, there will be some improvement in your condition by the fourth or fifth treatment, if not earlier (you may, of course, start to feel better after the first session). Once you do start to improve, it is very important to keep up with the treatment until the acupuncturist says you can stop. This goes back to the business of balancing energies. The first few treatments will start Chi flowing normally again, but if treatment is not continued you can easily relapse, leaving you just as unbalanced but perhaps with different symptoms.

Treatment can take a long time; homeopaths say that returning a patient completely to normal takes, on average, one month for every year that he has been ill. So it can be expensive. If there appear to be several equally well-qualified acupuncturists near you, there is no harm in asking what they charge before making an appointment. You may be surprised at the difference in prices. As far as ear studs are concerned, I have heard of two acupuncturists working within twenty miles of each other, one of whom was charging more than ten times as much as the other for the insertion of an ear stud.

And, if it is an ear stud that you want, inquire whether the acupuncturist will check it regularly. Studs do need to be changed every two weeks, so avoid a practitioner who does not do this.

And now, having made your appointment, what can you expect when you go for treatment? Well, the acupuncturist will of course want to know about your present illness, your medical history, and your health in general. He will also examine your tongue, pulse, skin, and nails. And he will then make you comfortable on a couch or chair and insert the relevant needles.

Many people have become alarmed in recent times about the possibility of catching infections from unsterilized needles and, for this reason, prefer to see a doctor rather than a lay acupuncturist. However, all acupuncturists who have been trained at one of the recognized colleges will have been taught about the necessity for sterilizing needles. Nowadays most use disposable needles, which can be thrown away after a single use.

As the needles go in, you are likely to feel what is known as *needling sensation, radiation,* or, in Chinese, *deqi.* It can take a number of forms, often a dull ache, but sometimes a tingling. It should never be unpleasantly painful but can sometimes be quite fierce and may radiate a fairly long way. Sometimes patients feel slightly sick or light headed at this point, but it only lasts a second or two. Some patients experience a warm glow traveling along the length of the meridian; occasionally this is accompanied by a flush on the skin. It is important to keep as still as possible while the needles are in to avoid dislodging them.

After the treatment you may feel considerably better and often very relaxed. However, remember that you are not yet completely well. Sometimes a patient is so delighted at being relatively free of pain after a session of acupuncture that, despite warnings, he does more physical work than he should and sets himself back again. Having acupuncture treatment is like having a broken leg put into a cast. Once the plaster has set, the leg is comfortable and it may be possible, if you are careful, to walk with the aid of a crutch. However, the leg is still broken inside its plaster cast and needs to be allowed to rest in order to heal properly. In the same way, if you have been ill for some time, the initial acupuncture treatments will not heal you right away; they will only start energy flowing again. You must be patient and work with the treatment, no matter how exciting may be the prospect of doing things that were previously impossible.

Occasionally, after a session of acupuncture, a patient's symptoms may become a great deal worse. This, surprisingly, is a good sign. It also occurs in other therapies, such as homeopathy (where it is known as aggravation) and in energy healing (where it is called a healing reaction). It is always a sign that the patient is going to respond well to treatment, so it should be an encouragement to continue, not an indication to give up. The reaction usually lasts twenty-four hours or less and is often followed fairly quickly by a considerable improvement in the condition.

One thing that people always seem to note when they see a complementary practitioner is that he has far more time to give them than the average family doctor, who is usually rushing to get through a waiting room full of patients. A visit to a complementary practitioner is far more leisurely, with greater opportunity for asking questions about your health problems and the treatment being given. Some practitioners will make house calls for patients whose condition prevents them from getting to the office; if appropriate, you can ask about this when you first contact an acupuncturist.

At present little use is made of acupuncture in place of anesthesia, except in the Far East. However, since a number of anesthetists use acupuncture in their pain clinics, it is possible that some might be willing to use it for suitable patients having minor operations. It is certainly possible to have acupuncture instead of painkillers during childbirth, which has the great advantage that there is no risk to the baby. For a mother who is having a home birth, arrangements can be made with an acupuncturist of her choice and with the midwife who is to do the delivery. In the case of a hospital birth, however, the obstetrician will have to give his permission for an acupuncturist to treat the patient while she is in the labor room.

One great advantage of acupuncture and other holistic therapies is that, fairly early on in the treatment, you are likely to start feeling better—possibly even before the symptoms of your disease start to improve. (A case in point was Mr. J. A., whose case was described in chapter 7.) The ultimate aim of acupuncture is to bring you into perfect balance. It is this balance, and not just an absence of disease, that constitutes good health.

Resources

American College of Acupuncture and Oriental Medicine
9100 Park West Drive
Houston, TX 77063
Telephone: 713-780-9777 • Fax: 713-781-5781
E-mail: webmaster@acaom.edu
Website: www.acaom.edu

South Baylo University
1126 N. Brookhurst St.
Anaheim, CA 92801-1706
Telephone: 714-533-1495 • Fax: 714-533-6040
E-mail: admin@southbaylo.edu
Website: www.southbaylo.edu

Florida College of Integrative Medicine
7100 Lake Ellenor Drive
Orlando, Florida 32809
Telephone: 407-888-8689 • Fax: 407-888-8211
E-mail: info@acupunctureschool.com
Website: www.fcim.edu

International College of Traditional Chinese Medicine of Vancouver
Suite 201, 1508 W. Broadway
Vancouver, B.C.
Canada V6J 1W8
Telephone: 604-731-2926 • Fax: 604-731-2964
E-mail: info@tcmcollege.com
Website: www.tcmcollege.com

The Council of Colleges of Acupuncture and Oriental Medicine (CCAOM)
3909 National Drive, Suite 125
Burtonsville, MD 20866
Telephone: 301-476-7790
Fax: 301-476-7792
Website: www.ccaom.org

The CCAOM was formed in 1982 to advance the status of acupuncture and Oriental medicine in the United States. It established the Accreditation Commission for Acupuncture and Oriental Medicine(ACAOM) to evaluate residential programs of acupuncture and Oriental medicine. It is recognized by the U.S. Department of Education and the Council on Higher Education Accreditation.

British Acupuncture Council
63 Jeddo Road
London W12 9HQ
Telephone: 020 8735 0400
Fax: 020 8735 0404
Website: www.acupuncture.org.uk

Index

Note: *Italic* page numbers indicate illustrations.

in the Sanjiao meridian, 52–53
in the Small Intestine meridian, 48–49
in the Spleen meridian, 46–47
in the Stomach meridian, 45–46
pulse diagnosis of, 95, 96
shingles, 40
six external factors
as causes of disease, 69–75
sleeping habits, 102
See also wind, cold, damp, dryness,
heat, summer heat
summer heat, 73–75
affecting the bladder, 91
affecting the gall bladder, 89
affecting the large intestine, 90
causing heatstroke, 144
See also six external factors

tinnitus, 136–37
tongue diagnosis, 96–100
coating of the tongue, 97–98
condition of the tongue, 99–100
pale tongue, 97
purple tongue, 97
purplish red tongue, 97
red tongue, 97
Treatment of the Seven Dragons, 163–64

urination, 49, 88
urticaria, 135

vital force, 3, 32, 82, 166–67. *See also* Chi

Western medicine, methods of treatment
by, 1, 2, 28, 29–30, 114–15
wind, 70–71, 100
affecting the liver, 85

affecting the lung, 87
reflected in tongue diagnosis, 98
See also six external factors
wrist drop, 158

Yellow Emperor, 6–7
Yellow Emperor's Classic of Internal
Medicine. *See* acupuncture, books
on, *Nei Ching*
yin and yang, 34–38, 80
and anger, 75
formation of excess yang, 122
in cold-related conditions, 71–72
in damp-related conditions, 72
in dryness-related conditions, 73
in heat-related conditions, 73–74
in pulse diagnosis, 95–96
in wind-related conditions, 70
meridians, 42–43, 44, 45, 52, 54
of the heart, 83–84
of the kidney, 88–89
of the lung, 87
of the stomach, 90

zang-fu organs, 83
bladder, 91
gallbladder, 89
heart, 83–84
kidney, 88–89
large intestine, 90
liver, 84–85
lung, 86–87
pericardium, 89
small intestine, 83
spleen, 85–86
stomach, 89–90B

BOOKS OF RELATED INTEREST

Acupuncture Energetics
A Workbook for Diagnostics and Treatment
by Mark Seem, Ph.D.

Acupuncture Imaging
Perceiving the Energy Pathways of the Body
by Mark D. Seem, Ph.D., DIPL. AC. (NCAA)

The Acupuncture Treatment of Pain
Safe and Effective Methods for Using Acupuncture in Pain Relief
by Leon Chaitow, D.O., N.D.

Acupressure Taping
The Practice of Acutaping for Chronic Pain and Injuries
by Hans-Ulrich Hecker, M.D., and Kay Liebchen, M.D.

The Acupressure Atlas
by Bernard C. Kolster, M.D., and Astrid Waskowiak, M.D.

Acupressure Techniques
A Self-Help Guide
by Julian Kenyon, M.D.

Trigger Point Therapy for Myofascial Pain
The Practice of Informed Touch
by Donna Finando, L.Ac., L.M.T., and Steven Finando, Ph.D., L.Ac.

Total Reflexology
The Reflex Points for Physical, Emotional, and Psychological Healing
by Martine Faure-Alderson, D.O.

Inner Traditions • Bear & Company
P.O. Box 388
Rochester, VT 05767
1-800-246-8648
www.InnerTraditions.com

Or contact your local bookseller